A supervision model

Lilja Cajvert

A supervision model

From initial interview to completed
supervision assignment

The book was first published in Swedish as
Handledning – Från intervju till avslutat uppdrag
ISBN 978-91-44-12785-9, Studentlitteratur 2019
A draft translation was prepared by Magnus Koch and later revised by P-O Aston.

© 2023 Lilja Cajvert
Publisher: BoD – Books on Demand, Stockholm, Sweden
Printer: BoD – Books on Demand, Norderstedt, Germany
ISBN: 978-91-8080-263-5

To my grandchildren Julia, Linnéa, Ellen and Oscar
Carry on being playful and creative.

Lilja Cajvert

Contents

Preface

Today there is a great deal of literature on supervision, in Swedish and in other languages. My own library at home contains around 80 titles on the subject, which is just a selection of what is currently available on the market. Aside from these books I have many articles, dissertations, essays etc. The sources are theoretical, describing various supervision models and methods. Many of the authors of these books are themselves supervisors, describing their own experiences of supervision.

This book is unlike other books on supervision. It describes the model I am using as a supervisor, how it was developed and how I apply it in practice. I've been using my own notes since 1983 and continuous evaluations of my supervision groups assessing what I'm doing and potential benefits for the supervisees: What should I continue to do as supervisor? What requires further development? What should be deleted or modified?

I usually ask the supervisees for feedback – this is something that we do together. In such evaluations participants often early on remark that my way of asking questions is somewhat unusual. For example:

"You question. You act differently. You want to understand, and I must reassess my thoughts and feelings and respond on a deeper level than simply saying how I am thinking and feeling. You force me to think harder. To reflect. Not just to talk. It's tough while it's going on. You don't give up. I must really think – by reconsidering once more new perspectives open. In that way it's uplifting, evolving. But it's tough. Please continue to be yourself and do ask questions."

Listening to such narratives for 40 years has also affected me. I was forced to think and reflect to understand what I was doing. To understand my intentions, how and why. These ongoing reflections on my own experiences and the subsequent increased awareness have led to a continuous development of my model of supervision. I've realised that there is a rationale for what I am doing, a common thread running through my work, a thought, a theoretical idea. I am not guided by chance or impulse. Supervision is a complex professional task, too liable, demanding and solitary to be undertaken without reflection and awareness of each step to be taken. We must know what we're doing, why and to what purpose.

Reflecting on my experiences and having an awareness of what I do, have formed the basis for the development of my own style of supervision and the model outlined in this book. This book presents just that. I describe what I do as a supervisor and how. It contains many citations from supervisees who over the years and in a variety of supervisory contexts have commented my work as a supervisor.

What has shaped my model of supervision?

Several factors in combination have been essential to the development of the model:
- my interest in and curiosity about the dynamic processes within supervision groups
- my curiosity about precisely what I'm doing during the supervision sessions
- the ongoing reflections and evaluations I undertook together with the supervisees
- the process of supervision of my own supervision.

Based on these experiences I developed models also described in the book:
- a model for presenting myself prior to a new assignment.
- a model for working with unconscious processes in dialogue with the supervisee.
- a model for working with parallel processes.

Why do I author this book – to whom?

The book describes a model of supervision from the introduction at an interview with a presumptive group to the completion of a supervision assignment. For beginners and for students enrolled in a variety of courses in supervision the book may be a source of knowledge on how you may shape and develop a supervision model.

The book should inspire other supervisors to clarify their own style of supervision, to reflect on the aims of their supervision assignment. To reflect on their own experiences and the way in which these direct and shape them as supervisors, in what they are doing or not doing during the assignment. An experienced supervisor may ask: What can we do ourselves and how? We could be brave and ask the supervisees what they have benefited from for their own development in the supervision, and how did the supervision concretely help in their own development as professionals. For readers with greater experience as supervisors some areas described will be familiar and others less so. In any case, the book may serve as a basis for the conscious articulation of and reflection on one's own style and experiences, to gain insight into what you can do and what might be beyond the scope of the supervision.

The book also addresses the supervisees in supervisory groups. The supervisory sessions may inspire the participants to reflect on what they want to get from their supervision. Becoming aware of the impact of what we do on the individuals with whom we are working is an essential aspect of professional practice, whether you are engaged in treatment, as physicians and teachers, in psychotherapy or in mentoring. In meeting with others who are seeking our help and relying on our practice an attitude of reflection and awareness is needed – we must be conscious of the impact of our own participation and its bearing on a meeting, in establishing a relationship – but also, we must reflect on the aims and outcome of what we're doing.

Reading of other people's experiences of supervision and the way supervisors position themselves in the pursuit of an assignment inspires us to consider what we wish to take home from our own supervision. From a participant's point of view: What expectations do we have of the supervision, both as individuals and as a group? What approach should the supervision take to benefit your own professional development? Are you prepared to reflect on your own experiences and what is happening when you meet clients or colleagues? How are you contributing to what is achieved or not achieved? Do you want to get a lot of questions to understand and challenge yourself, or is the supervision more of an opportunity for rest and relaxation? For a manager who is budgeting supervision, this book may inspire to get more information about how supervision is perceived by the supervisees. The book may also stimulate leaders to find appropriate ways to be involved in a group supervision of their employees. What are the desired outcomes for the group? What sort of contact is required with the supervisor and to what purpose? The book may also help deciding whether the group is better off without the manager's involvement, perhaps not knowing anything of the content or the process, or even not being present at an evaluation. Perhaps no contact is needed after signing the contract. I've led many groups in which I have had no contact with the manager or even knowing who that person is. I always offer an opportunity, but it is the management who has the last word.

Thanks

Writing is a lonely job. It is at times filled with pressure and anxiety as it applies to the creative process. You get writer's block, or is stuck on a line of thought, and it is also hard to know when to stop writing. Whenever I have found myself in this position I have had the support of my publisher Johan Lindgren. Without his support there would be no book. A big thanks, Johan. Thanks Anna Åström and Eva Broberg for your input and skill in making sure that the original edition in Swedish was clear and easy to read. Thanks to Magnus Koch and P-O Aston for a sensitive translation.

My sincere thanks to all the professional persons I have supervised over the course of more than four decades. Without your opinions and feedback on what I do and do not do, I would not have been able to develop my supervision style presented in this book.

Lilja Cajvert
January 2023
lilja.cajvert@icloud.com

Introduction

What is supervision?

According to current literature supervision provides tools to professionals to create preconditions for further use and development of their competence. The goal of supervision is to develop a "professional identity", the specific readiness and capacity to use oneself as a tool in the work with clients (Bernler & Johnsson, 1985; Cajvert, 1998, 2013; Gordan, 1998; Hawkins & Shohet, 2000). Supervision may be defined as a process of learning. Anderson and Goolishian (1992) argue that the purpose of supervision is to build a creative dialogue in which new knowledge and insights encourage seeing the work with a client from as many perspectives as possible. The values and attitudes of the supervisee in relation to the ongoing issue should be a focus of the supervision (Cajvert, 1998). The key to learning in supervision is to reflect on your own experiences while carrying out your professional activities (Van Kessel and Haan , 1993). Supervision is in this sense an ongoing process of life-long learning for the professional (Žorga, 2002) and through the supervision the supervisor and supervisee have a continuous dialogue from which both can learn (Cajvert, 2013).

Bernard and Goodyear (2009) use the term "supervision as a three-person-system" to describe the relationships involved. Supervision involves two separate relations *client-therapist* and *therapist-supervisor*. The therapist is the person common to both relations and functions as a channel for both information and processes that involve both relations.

In my view, supervision is the supervisee's creative space, where all thoughts may be spoken out loud and where there is an opportunity to share experiences and ideas through mutual dialogue between the supervisee and supervisor. Dialogue and reflection increase the supervisees' self-understanding and provide opportunities to process their own experiences. The supervision is aimed at professional development within a given field and becomes a learning process, in which the supervisees may integrate theory and practice, and in an efficient and conscious way utilise their expertise within their professional work.

Through supervision the collective capacity of the group is utilized, and supervision becomes a quality assurance, benefiting the organisation, the client and the supervisees.

Process supervision help us understanding relationships and processes that we encounter as professionals, an opportunity for reflection on what we do in our encounters with clients, to develop our general competence rather than specific skills. Process supervision has an overall focus, and the supervisee becomes part of the treatment or pedagogic system she or he belongs to. It is a step towards greater professionalism. The group and supervisor may together question all that is in focus, view it from several perspectives before embarking on the next step in the process. Supervision is a creative process carried out within different theories and models. It is life-long learning.

A couple of participants in supervision groups:

"Supervision is a space in which I can be myself. I can raise questions on how I feel in any situation. For example, not what to do when giving a client a negative decision, but more related to how it feels to communicate such a decision. To have the opportunity once a month to reflect on myself and my own experiences."

"I have high expectations of the supervision. To gain an understanding of why I react as I do in certain cases. Gaining new insights. Helping me to develop."

Agreements

There are various agreements within the framework of a supervisor assignment. Some of these are written as a formal agreement, while others are more flexible, often oral, pertaining to day-to-day activities during the supervision.

A written contract is often established between a purchasing office and the supervisor, where price and content are agreed.

An agreement is also signed between the supervisor and the leader of the supervision group, stating the conditions of the supervision: timetable, scope, rules if the supervision is not done, the leader's expectations of the supervision as well as other formal details like invoicing.

Most agreements usually orally negotiated between the supervisor and the leader of the supervision group concern mutual expectations of the supervision in terms of activities, openness, and respect. How should conflicts be resolved and how will the supervisor respond to participants who are either very silent, or very talkative. Furthermore, confidentiality is discussed making sure what is raised during supervision is not disclosed.

A mandate is an agreement even if it is not explicitly stated. If the supervisor at the interview introduces a style and method of supervision and the group chooses to work with that supervisor there is an implicit agreement, or mandate. In my own supervision this entails that the group members are willing to be the focus of attention, can be supervised and they also commit to being active. Above all the mandate allows me as supervisor to work with unconscious processes using a model I have developed, but also to work with other methods I have presented at the interview.

Agreements should be flexible and can be changed according to the needs of the group. A clear mandate at the beginning of the assignment is a necessary condition to create a working alliance and relationship with the group members. The agreement clarifies the purpose of the supervision.

My approach in the book

The book is divided into eight parts, corresponding to what I present in the initial interview with a supervision group and how I present my supervision model.

Synopsis – first interview with a supervision group

The table on the following pages is a summary of the presentation of my model I use in a first interview.

The first interview with a supervision group

Framework of the meeting
- Who participates in the meeting?
- How much time do we have?
- The supervisor interviews the participants and/or the participants interviews the supervisor.

Comment The supervisor and each group select the form that this meeting will take.

Presentation of each participant
- Name
- Education, professional experience, current position, and area of work
- Experience of supervision, positive and less positive
- Expectation of the supervision
- Expectations on the group
- Expectations on yourself
- Expectations on the supervisor

Presentation of the supervisor and the supervisor's model (my own presentation)
- My view of supervision
- My theoretical basis
- What tools do I use in the supervision?
- The importance of all participants being in focus during the supervision sessions
- Short description of the supervision process and my own attitude:
- First, a short lecture on interactive processes and how to work with them
  - What is the purpose of my questions, in the spirit of Socrates and Wittgenstein?
  - How the supervision session usually develops
  - Importance of avoiding advice and suggestions to the supervisee
  - Working as "if this was my client, I would…" derived from Montague Ullman's model on understanding the language of dreams adapted to supervision work
  - What I don't do in supervision
  - My wish to establish contact with the group leader and to what purpose
- Review and evaluation during supervision. How, when and why?
  How do we terminate the supervision?
  My strengths and difficulties in supervision
  Meta-supervision
Preconditions
- Who will participate in the supervision?
- How many supervision sessions per term?
- How long is each session?
- Where will the supervision take place?
- Cost per supervision session

- Is supervision mandatory or voluntary?
- What is said in the supervision is not shared with others, or the management
- Who volunteers to be contact person for administrative matters with the supervisor?
- Who participates in the meeting?
- How much time do we have?
- The supervisor interviews the participants and/or the participants interviews the supervisor.
- What expectations do I have of the supervision group and of the supervisee
  - Each participant is willing to be in focus and to be supervised
  - any participant can raise any question without being judged, condemned or questioned
  - if anyone has an issue with the supervision, this will be evaluated and tackled during the supervision

As supervisor it is my role, assignment, and function to:
- Maintain structure
- Pave the way for the agreed goals of the supervision
- Contribute to creating a working alliance, a safe space and constructive climate in the group
- Endorse and challenge
- Support and offer advice if requested
- Engage all participants in what is going on professionally and in the supervision group
- Stimulate and initiate further professional development
- Offer theoretical analysis and explanation when required
- Be a model

Focus during the supervision
- Client-oriented: who is the client?
- Task-oriented: what is the issue?
- Method-oriented: how do we work, how do we progress, what is our attitude, which method?
- Theme-oriented: different themes are raised in the supervision relating to work, to the group in focus, to the organization, to the leadership etc.
- Theoretical analysis and explanation
- Process-oriented supervision at different levels, with focus on:
  The supervisee's own professional process, thoughts and feelings
  Interaction between client and supervisee
  Interaction supervisee – supervisor
  Interaction supervisee – other participants in the group or with colleagues
  Interaction supervisor – supervision group
  Interaction within the group at the place of work or during the supervision

1. The Interview

The supervisor

How is a supervision assignment established? Usually a manager, or a person who is part of a management team, contacts a supervisor asking if she/he is available to supervise a group of workers. If the supervisor is interested and available, a time is suggested for an interview.

The interview for a potential supervision assignment can take a variety of forms. It depends on who is doing the interview, who is present during the interview, and what one wants to know about the supervisor and his/her supervision model. Here is a description of how the supervisor might present himself/herself at an interview with a potential supervision group based on my own general technique.

The setting of the interview may vary:
- The whole group is present
- Some individuals are representatives for the group, being assigned by the group to interview a few supervisors
- The manager interviews initially and on a later occasion the whole group
- Only the manager interviews the supervisor
- Less commonly the group does not interview the supervisor at all, but relies on the description in an ad and prior knowledge of the supervisor.

The persons present at the interview influence the content and questions that the supervisor might ask of the group. The purpose of the interview should be to gain a sufficiently clear idea of one another to be ready to begin a supervision together.

Information prior to the interview

Sometimes a group might request a short introduction from the supervisor prior to the interview (see text in the box below); I write a brief note on what I consider important for the group to know about my experience of supervision, my theoretical basis and my supervision method. Furthermore, it's important for them to know how I perceive my own and their duties, and our shared responsibility.

At the end I give some references from recently completed and ongoing supervisions. Since I'm developing and changing as a supervisor and references from earlier work are no longer representative. I forward the same text if the group has selected me as supervisor prior to an interview with their manager:

Lilja Cajvert, social worker, Ph.lic., lecturer in social work, reg. psychotherapist and supervisor

Experience of supervision
I have been working as a supervisor in Sweden since 1983, for several government and administrative authorities, in therapeutic and other professional areas such as social services, geriatric care, healthcare, childcare, fostering services, penal establishments, institutional care, schools, family law, institutions for migrant minors etc.

Other relevant experience
I have been a teacher, worked as a supervisor and been an academic examiner in university social studies departments, M.A. programs, supervisor training and psychotherapy courses. Since 2015, I have run courses of supervision education in psychosocial work at the Department of Social Work, Göteborg University. I have also since 1998 periodically undertaken supervision internationally in post-conflict countries. Between 2012–2015 I took part in an EU project that developed a European standard dictionary and matrix of competence for supervision and coaching within Europe.

Basic theory and supervision method
My theoretical basis is in object-relations theory and attachment theory emphasising the importance of relationships for the development of the individual, and systems theory that stresses a holistic view seeing everyone within her social context. My general attitude derives from Wittgenstein, Socrates and Buber's philosophy, as well as phenomenology. I utilise a variety of supervision theories and supervision methods to develop the dialogue and process within the framework of process supervision, method supervision and task or case supervision. Within supervision the supervisees are given the opportunity to reflect upon and question their task and what is being demanded of them, to use their resources and knowledge/methods and in this way broaden their views and see what unfolds in a variety of perspectives. I work innovatively

and develop methods and techniques that I apply practically in supervision and continue to develop on a theoretical level in my texts.

Focus during supervision

Within supervision you can raise any issue you are struggling with in your work, to find the best solution to work professionally with your clients. All group members are active and participate. The person in focus formulates with my help a supervision question that she at the end of the supervision session wish to see resolved, and then decide how to proceed. Everyone in the group and myself as the supervisor contributes to resolving the question from a range of perspectives.

The supervisee in focus chooses with my help as supervisor how she wish to use the group's resources. One can choose techniques like *'reflecting team'*, *'as if'*, *'role play'*, *'taping'*, and so on. The group members can also offer suggestions and advice on what they would have done given the situation and facing the question as described by the supervisee. Thus, they get counsel on their ideas while the supervisee in focus observes, and finally chooses "the path" which she herself wants to adopt. For her it is a case of learning and broadening her point of view through someone else's perspective.

If the supervisee wishes to focus the feeling generated in relation to a client, I have developed working methods to decide which interactive processes have the greatest impact, or what, on a personal level, seems to be activated in working with the client. My experience is that everyone develops professionally and on a personal level after a few seasons of this supervision model.

At some point during the supervision period, after a year, we invite the manager to attend our evaluation of the supervision. The group and I decide what is important to share with the manager regarding the development of the supervision, and how we should proceed.

Agreements

As supervisor I am tasked with helping the supervisee to formulate a supervision question or to understand what help he/she would like to get. My responsibility is to maintain the structure and a common thread, to make sure that all are active and that all are in focus at some point. The supervisee must be willing to be supervised, to be open to supervision and feedback, and in turn to give feedback. It's important that all group members remain active and interested during the supervision even when they are not in focus.

From the group members I expect commitment and that they are prepared to communicate if they are not satisfied with the supervision, or with me as supervisor. If we bring up an issue early there's a chance for us to put it right instead of someone remaining dissatisfied for a long time, or not attending the supervision, or wanting to terminate it.

References
I usually offer completed and ongoing references, with contact details to those persons who have consented to be referees. Usually, I cite two or three persons and give a few relevant publications

Interview with a potential supervision group

The interview may begin with the group participants and the supervisor deciding on the structure of the interview, and on who will be responsible for maintaining the structure. Preferably, the supervisor is given the responsibility. The group may then get an initial impression of the supervisor's way of leading the dialogue and process, how she maintains the structure and interest of the group.

As the interview usually lasts for an hour "everything" that needs to be said can be covered, but concisely. Furthermore, the group may have received a short introduction by email (see my introduction above).

The first interview with a potential supervision group may be divided into the following stages: introduction, expectations, and the setting of the supervision. This provides an opportunity for a mutual exchange of information, on the views and expectations of the supervision.

If the group is interviewing me, based on questions circulated in advance, I want to explain at the end of the interview what remains to be covered: matters that I wish to communicate about my supervision style and the theoretical basis of my work. Regardless of the model chosen I want the group first to present themselves along with their expectations of supervision. Thus, my intention is that the group and its individuals should not be influenced by my view of supervision, or my presentation of the supervision model.

Presentation of the supervision model

As supervisor you may for instance begin by briefly describing your experience as a supervisor and your educational background. Then, you can describe the theoretical basis of your work, your view of human beings, therapeutics and supervision. You might begin with how you work with supervision, how the process of supervision functions during sessions and the methods used. I personally also briefly describe how I handle interactive processes during the supervision. I usually share what other groups have commented on my supervision and about me as a supervisor during the evaluations, including what seems most satisfactory, what should be continued or further developed, and what should be changed.

How to present your experience of work?

How can we share experiences of work and supervision without sounding like presenting a CV? Relate only as much you believe to be relevant to the present supervision and the present group. I usually say that I have a long experience of supervision – since 1983 – that I have supervised different types of groups and professions within the social services, care professions and welfare, schools etc. If I haven't had any experience of giving supervision to enterprises like the present one, I mention this, but also state that I'm keen to learn something new.

Theoretical basis and how to use theories in supervision

Theories and theoretical terms are explained during the supervision in various ways. Sometimes it's necessary to abstract or distance yourself from what occurs between the supervisee and client, or the supervisee and supervisor. To clarify or explain what is happening from a theoretical point of view is giving a supervisee the chance to integrate theoretical knowledge with practical experience. I also use theory in circumstances when I'm clarifying and explaining my questions, my interventions, or my actions.

Each new supervision assignment begins with a lecture. It includes theoretical explanations and definitions of certain psychodynamic concepts and processes occurring in the meeting between the client and supervisee and/or the supervisee and supervisor. In any meeting we are affected by one another, and by our earlier life and work experiences. Unconscious processes can only be discovered as they occur and can only be understood retrospectively.

In the field of psychodynamic psychotherapy, I am drawn to object relation theory and attachment theory, with its emphasis on the importance of relationships for the development of the individual.

I also use a systems-theoretical framework, a holistic approach that stresses the individual within a social context, as an added strategy for what seems to be lacking in psychodynamic theory. A systemic approach (Wonnacott 2012) is useful in analysing how different parts and the whole connect, how they influence and in turn are influenced by each other.

As professionals and supervisors, we are part of the dynamic process, it affects us, and we affect it. We are part of a social structure and are subject to different conditions and our capacity for action varies. This is true for the client as well as for the supervisee and the supervisor.

Philosophy is my source of inspiration to help the supervisee to find their own answers and methods, and to better understand their actions. From Wittgenstein's philosophy (1978) I take a basic understanding of the importance of language in dialogue. Wittgenstein helps us to understand the way in which language and behaviour are intimately connected. We learn the meaning of words and what they may signify in a variety of contexts. Therefore, it's important to learn the meaning of words in the sense that they are used by others and not only from my own interpretation and what the words may mean to me. This attitude leads me to ask what certain words might signify for the other person to better understand the other person's use of a word and not assuming a meaning according to my own usage and understanding. When for example someone says he is angry, in pain, upset, disappointed and so on, I can understand what these words signify in contexts I have used these words myself when angry, in pain, upset or disappointed, but that doesn't mean they have the same meaning for the supervisee as for myself. That is why I am asking the supervisee to clarify the meaning of words awaking strong feelings that seem to hinder his professional work. By asking how a person responds and acts when angry, in pain, upset or disappointed, in case these words have been used we explore and enrich the conversation.

Socratic questioning is useful to develop the dialogue and help the supervisee to articulate knowledge and thoughts he is full of. The supervisee is guided through dialogue and questions to articulate his own thoughts and ideas prior to other group members and myself as supervisor, share our own thoughts and ideas on the theme in focus.

Buber's philosophy (1990) on closeness and distance enriches my understanding of an approach in which both the Thou–I and Thou–It relationships fit in the therapeutic and supervising situation. To be able to help you must have a relationship and be part of this 'Thou–I' relation. When the supervisee in the supervision needs to assess, reflect and communicate on his client he is in a I–It relationship and maintains distance and "sees" the other from a different perspective.

Phenomenology (Kordeš, 2008) is applicable when I and the supervision group are observing our experience of the ongoing relationship and of what is occurring in the supervision, without immediately beginning to analyse and theorise. In a way, we would like to access the meaning of our experience as it occurs to us in the moment, against the background of what happened and was shown in action. Thus, we are in the moment and 'in the world' instead of analysing it. Phenomenology is useful especially when working with parallel processes during the supervision, in which I am a part of these processes by my feelings and thoughts that were raised and became an obstacle for me in my role as supervisor, in the same way that parallel processes are obstacles for the supervisee in meeting with the client presented during the supervision.

Why asking in-depth follow-up questions?

Asking in-depth questions is a central feature of my supervision model. However, the questions have no obvious answer. Using questions, I want to encourage the supervisee's inner dialogue, to help her reflect on the reasons why she acts as she does. Hopefully, the supervisee gains a greater understanding of her own involvement in the processes that arise between herself and a client. The questions should also raise an awareness and questioning of who's frame of reference is guiding the work – is it that of the client, or one's own.

The technique of working with questions has helped many therapists in their relationships with clients. Through experience-based learning the therapists acquire knowledge on how to use questions as a tool in their work.

My ambition is to facilitate a reflective approach in the supervision to explore ways in which we put questions to clients. What is the purpose of these questions and how do we utilise the answers? In what way does the therapist asking questions take the process forward and so on.

Already during the interview, I am asking in-depth questions to demonstrate how this may be done in the context of supervision.

As already mentioned, it's common for supervisees at the evaluation, and sometimes at the beginning of the supervision, to say that they're not used to my way of asking questions. To paraphrase one supervisee:

"You want to understand, and I must re-run my thoughts and feelings. It's on a deeper level than simply saying how I think and feel. It's tough while it's going on. You don't give up. I must think and as I again run it over, new perspectives open. In that way it's uplifting, progress is being made. But it's tough. Please continue as you've been doing and keep asking those questions."

Åsa Nilsonne (2017) argues: "Even if it's hard and sometimes impossible to find answers, raising questions is helpful. It's helpful to be met with goodwill and respect as I try to be less confused." (p. 154)

If problems arise

In the case problems can't be solved and the supervision does not remain a worthwhile and creative space, the group members and supervisor may decide to end the supervision assignment earlier than planned.

Evaluation of the supervision

Evaluation may be undertaken on different occasions and for different purposes. After each session of supervision, it is done to jointly sum up and reflect on the current process. If difficulties have arisen during the supervision, it becomes especially important to evaluate. What were the expectations? How did things turn out? How are we to continue? What should we change?

I usually come to an agreement with the manager and the group that the manager attends an evaluation, at least once a year. The group and I list on a board the themes and issues we have dealt with in the supervision. At the end of the session the manager participates for an hour. We may then have a dialogue about the supervision so far and the areas that the group and the manager wish us to focus during the next period.

My strengths and difficulties

One of my strengths is the ability to maintain a common thread within the theme which we have in focus and that we are currently discussing. I wait for the answers to my questions or make a note that I have not had any answers before continuing with another theme. The supervisees value my commitment to and curiosity about what goes on between the professional and client, or the professional and myself, likewise they value my mental presence. I'm not afraid of conflict and am able to take criticism, but I'm also bold enough to point out inconsistencies when clearly shown in the supervision.

I prepare myself before each meeting of the group, especially when I have noticed the group's or my own disappointment with the supervision process. I don't have a problem asking even when it's a difficult situation and I share my own weaknesses as I become aware of them.

At the interview I usually discuss my own difficulties as a supervisor, both those of which I have been aware for a long time and those that have been pointed out to me at various evaluations. The supervisees have made me realise that I am sometimes too fast in asking questions or that I sometimes ask too many and "too difficult" questions. Sometimes group members can feel under pressure to appear clever, whether in answering my questions or in formulating new supervision questions. They want me to repeat, even if it may be one time too many, that the supervision question need not be formulated in advance, and also, I can help drafting the question.

Occasionally I may find it difficult to discover in time when someone in the group competes with me in my role as supervisor, or when group members compete with one another. Once I have become aware of such a competition, I have no trouble raising the matter with the person concerned during the supervision.

Supervision of the supervisor – meta supervision

As a supervisor I am affected by the processes in supervision groups or by counter-transference responses occurring in relation to the supervisees. When necessary, I am getting supervision on the supervision, in which case I am in focus in the same way as the supervisees are during the supervision that I'm giving. I then have the opportunity for dialogue, assistance, and support.

Group members

The group members introduce themselves with their name, educational background and briefly relate their work experiences focusing on their current employment. What position does the individual have within the organisation? The discussion also covers previous experiences of supervision, both positive ones and less so. What are the expectations of the supervision, of the group, of themselves and the role of the supervisor? In the following section some cited answers may be representative of many others.

Group members experience of supervision

Why should you raise the question of earlier experiences of supervision? To find out what the group appreciates in supervision. But it's just as interesting to learn of less positive experiences in order not to repeat them, or to try to identify them early in the process. It's clear that certain processes may recur, and the questions help the supervisor to find solutions in time.

Good experiences

Most groups have positive experiences of supervision. Such experiences may be related to the atmosphere in the group, or that the supervision has been useful, or that the process adopted by the supervisor was satisfactory. When the group for example mentions a positive atmosphere the supervisor at the interview may probe more deeply and ask: "What is a positive atmosphere? How did that show in your group?"

Some examples of how groups have responded to such questions:

Positive atmosphere in the group is when it's possible to: "Feel safe in the group" or "Everyone is participating", "When everyone can ponder his question in a caring environment", "When there's room for pause, to be able to think: What am I doing?". "The supervision was fine because we didn't have a boss."

The most common answer to the question "What makes the supervision a *fruitful undertaking?*" is "I got something to take home". It may be a feeling of relief, a feeling of being energised, or that we've been able to talk to each other in a way for which there is neither time nor inclination during working hours. To be able to pause and reflect.

Good supervision entails that we: "Gain something positive from the group – and leave the supervision somewhat wiser", "Hear a different perspective which my mind would not otherwise have considered, both from the supervisor and the others in the group", "When the supervisor dares to ask questions. Is interested in earnest", "When I can talk about various difficult issues that are hard to handle".

It's not unusual for the group to raise the importance of the supervisor in creating a positive experience of supervision. The manner of the supervisor, the materials she uses and the way in which the participation of the whole group is facilitated, all of these are important. To get help resolving one's supervision question, or by resolving anxiety provides an experience of a positive supervision.

"It's useful when a supervisor is attentive to our thoughts, opens up, using a wide perspective", "The supervisor took our worries seriously", "The supervisor uses a range of images", "Enable others to participate", "Feel that the supervisor is listening", "When the supervisor is active. When the supervisor directs [...] how it's to be done", "To be helped by the supervisor to close what I need to close down".

Less positive experiences

Often some group members raise issues in the supervision of which they are dissatisfied. For example, when the supervisor talks too much about herself, even about private matters. In such cases I usually ask:

"What does private matters mean? Please exemplify? How should I find out that I've been too private? How would you like us to continue when such a situation arises, and you are dissatisfied? What part of my professional experiences would you like me to share?"

Less positive experiences of the supervision can also be viewed in relation to the atmosphere in the group, or when there is a lack of trust and honesty. Trust within the group is very important in making any supervision fruitful. Honesty is appreciated and when lacking the supervision is less satisfactory.

Some examples of what different groups might say:

"Less positive supervision happens when I don't feel trust in the group, when I feel challenged and respond defensively. Then I respond with 'reserved silence'", "Even worse when honesty is lacking, and this is not addressed "It can also lead to difficulties when there is tension between one person and the supervisor. This becomes a difficulty also for the group", "When you are offended by the supervisor", "When you are not participating, just sitting out the session", "When someone takes up all available supervision time and the rest of the group becomes an audience", "When the supervision feels like a coffee break", "When it's not working the problem is often in the group, not about the supervisor. What can the supervisor do in the case of a poor group atmosphere and group members feeling bad?".

Such statements are important to clarify – for example, the supervisor has to understand what may have been offensive and how she will find out that she is offending a participant and in what way. Or how the supervision appears when it is like a coffee break. Or how dishonesty might seem, and so on.

The group members are quite aware of what supervisor and type of supervision they don't want. It's as much about the supervisor's relationship with the group or the individual, as how the supervisor should not be.

"It's difficult when the supervisor doesn't see what is happening in the group", "Supervisors who would like to be like teachers and act as instructors and claim to know best give a negative experience. You don't want that type of supervisor", "When the supervisor complains and points out: 'oh what a difficult situation you're in'", "When the supervisor comes up with quick solutions, is focused on resolving everything and talks a lot herself, and the group has hardly a say", "When the supervisor comes up with readymade solutions: 'do this'", "When the supervisor does not intervene when the group fails and people start accusing one another", "When the supervisor isn't attentive to what is happening in the group", "When the supervisor takes over and wants to talk about her own experiences", "The supervisor doesn't care about the process of the supervisees", "When we don't have any issues to discuss and the supervisor is not prepared with an agenda for how we use the session time", "When everyone is silent and the supervisor doesn't help out", "When there is a lack of honesty and the situation is very emotional. The supervisor makes a note of this, but it isn't expressed", "When the supervisor is just teaching and want to appear smart. Lectures those who know best".

When group members discuss their experiences at the interview, I ask them what we should do if I as the supervisor find myself in any of the given situations. How will I find out about this in time so that we can change things together? My intention is to have a positive supervision, that I don't hurt or offend individuals or the group, but if it should happen, I want to be told.

When I at the interview ask the group members to expand on their statements and the significance of the words that they use, the group "becomes aware of" my method of asking questions, to probe more deeply into what is being said, and understand their understanding. I don't want to draw my own conclusions from my own understanding of the words they are using.

The supervisor may in such a situation already at the interview draw up a mini-contract on how they together can respond if something happens that the group or a group member is not happy with. This mini-contract entails the group members and the supervisor together to decide on how a future conflict may be resolved. For example, someone in the group may tell the supervisor, in case she does not pick it up, that the supervisee in focus feels pressed by the questions, or the group members believe that the supervisor is not on the same wavelength and that they are not getting the help they want.

I have experienced groups who at the interview brings up unsatisfactory matters in a previous supervision that are later repeated in our supervision. Then I can be prepared and won't immediately take the blame. One example: a group raised the fact that they were not satisfied with a previous supervision and terminated it as "it fizzled out". On my question about what happened in concrete terms and why "it fizzled out" they told me that for a long time they had no issues to raise, no one brought anything along to the supervision. After a few meetings this was repeated in our supervision. Time and again they had nothing to discuss. On one of these occasions the matter of what could be done was raised so that the supervision would not "fizzle out". We found a common strategy for what we could do. We found ourselves in this situation and agreed that it was the responsibility of both parties to help the process of the supervision to develop, instead of letting it fizzle out risking termination of the supervision.

To switch supervisor without seeing the pattern did not solve the problems of that group.

As a supervisor one must not concern oneself with finding out who were the group's previous supervisor(s). This is of no interest. Rather, it is about maintaining a professional ethical attitude and having respect for each other's supervision models.

For myself the question of "less positive experience" is useful and gives an idea of what I should be avoiding. Despite taking notes I am not always able to keep this in mind. I may miss noticing the process and forget revisiting my notes from the interview. As a supervisor I am part of the process created in the group.

From statements about positive and less positive experiences of supervision you may conclude that a supervisor will face several demands. When dissatisfaction occurs, it is unfortunately not always expressed. I'm convinced that most supervisors can support the group in creating a positive atmosphere and avoid behaving in a way the group does not want, if she realises the problem and tries to find a solution together with the group.

Group members' expectations

At the interview the supervisor will get to know what the group members expect of the supervision.

Expectations of the supervision

This means getting an idea of the expectations and hopes of each member of the group. To know this already at the start is a useful tool for the supervisor in deciding if she can fulfil the expectations of each member and the whole group. When every group member can express herself, everybody hears what the expectations are of each one, and how these correspond with others in the group.

I begin by asking about general expectations of the supervision but then broaden the question to ask what each participant expects of the group and of themselves. How might the group and they themselves contribute to the supervision so that it becomes the type of supervision that they request? The round on expectations is finished off with the question of what each one expects of me in my role as supervisor. Thereby I want to distinguish what are the expectations of the supervision in general, and of myself in my role as supervisor.

To have expectations of the supervision includes both what one would like to achieve for oneself and for the group. What will the supervision in this form yield? This is distinct from expectations on the supervisor's role which is more concerned with expectations on how the supervisor will proceed, and how she might orient herself to various situations or to certain processes within the group.

It is not always possible for the group members to tell what they expect of the supervision. If someone has no previous experience of supervision, the supervisor can put the same question in a different way:

"What would be enough rewarding for you to attend the supervision?"
- "Could you try to imagine what these meetings might offer you? What would you like us to do and talk about in the meetings?"

"What would qualify as meaningful discussions and dialogue for you, during such meetings?"

The purpose is to try to have the individual imagine and try to express her thoughts about the supervision meetings. This is also a way to show how the supervisor uses follow-up questions and doesn't leave individual members behind and simply move on or change focus when the reply is "I don't know", or "I haven't thought about it". As it is the first meeting with the group it's a matter of maintaining a balance between what and how the supervisor asks questions and gets for answers.

Already at the interview, I present the Socratic method and ask in-depth questions when someone says she don't know or hasn't thought. I want to show my interest in what that individual might say. I want to communicate the importance of everyone. All can contribute and in supervision everyone should be "on track". In-depth questions make it easier for those who reply "I don't know" to eventually say something about their expectations. But it may also be problematic for individuals and groups who do not wish to probe any further and view the supervision as an opportunity "to get out of work and have a rest". Then the questions can be difficult, and the supervisor seems demanding.

Expectations of the supervision depend on where you are in the process as a group and how accustomed group members are to receiving process supervision. Depending on the characteristics of the group and the enterprise, I separate expectations into several different categories:

A group dynamic and to get different perspectives
B on the tools and on the role of the supervisor
C challenges in the supervision
D difficulty of expressing expectations
E focus on oneself and on receiving feedback

A. Supervision offers an opportunity to group members to get to know one another and gain a variety of perspectives on their work. The expectation is to be accepted and to talk about difficult issues. Some voices:

"Listen to the thoughts and feelings of others and support one another", "There is a respectful listening to what is being said in the group. There is honesty and sharing. I allow myself not to know. The supervisor contributes valuable thoughts", "Listen to one another", "Respect each other's opinions", "working for better collaboration among us", "working to be a group", "Lift one's gaze, gain perspective", "Getting response from the supervisor and being able to speak in the group. Hear about the experiences of others", "Getting a gain from my working group and from colleagues. Know that the group is there. Method is more like a question in a task, for example who I should call. Process is more personal, such as how to connect with a patient that I don't like", "Get to speak about matters I can't handle at work", "A way to develop while working with a client and in the group", "A space where everything is acceptable", "Supervision should be a means to develop the work with the client and the group", "What transpires in the room is acknowledged in a permitting atmosphere. It's stable. Want to grow as a person", "I am able to talk about the importance of the organisation for my work", "Experiencing a calm not possible at work", "Permitted to discuss thoughts and feelings, to express oneself", "To be able to talk about difficult issues – hard to deal with at work".

B. Other expectations deal with how the supervisor should be and the wish to feel the supervision helping and offering an opportunity to look within yourself. Tools and techniques for dialogue are sought. Some voices:

"Supervision is like holding hands, maintaining structure and not having to worry about taking up too much space", "Matters are clear – what are we doing right now? The supervision should help us to find perspectives ourselves and contribute with knowledge", "Learn different techniques for a dialogue, get tools", "Learn methods for working with different people, use myself as a resource. Learn why I respond in the way I do", "To develop as a social worker and as a human being, see my own role in the situation", "Talk about tools, get advice", "I'm new in my role. Expect everyone to share their experiences. Not to feel alone".

C. Some group members expect a challenge from the supervision. It's a pathway to development. Through communication and teamwork, the group members learn and take part in each other's competences.

"We're here to challenge ourselves, get our group together. It's a very lonely job. A lot of expectations on us. I look forward to developing our competence together", "Everyone must be able to air their views and talk about what troubles them", "I'm open to talk about everything", "I want it to be okay to say things are tough", "Supervision is a development of competence".

D. Some people find it hard to express in words what it is they expect of supervision. It might be difficult to say anything at all, perhaps because previous experience of supervision is lacking. Some voices:

"Hard to express what it is", "Don't know, but it shouldn't feel worse than before the supervision", "Have no experience of supervision and don't know what to expect".

E. It's common for the supervisees to want to focus on themselves. To be observers of themselves, receiving feedback and trying to understand both the processes of which they are a part, their vocation and themselves. Some voices: "To be professional and realise what makes a professional social worker", "Get to know myself. Understand myself", "Become aware of myself and the processes in the families I am working with", "Want to be more stable, more secure", "To become aware of myself. Who am I?", "See my strengths", "Why do I sigh every time I get an email from that mother?", "Deal with what's weighing me down", "To understand the way I react", "To gain a deeper understanding of various matters", "Opportunity to work issues where I am stuck", "Why do I react the way I do in some meetings? To learn I'm not simply crazy", "What happens to me when I'm meeting the youths?", "To talk about a work situation and learn to understand myself better", "I'm a different social worker each case. The supervision helps me to see what is happening to me", "Something that helps me to develop in my role", "To get help on how to move on", "I have high expectations. To understand why I react the way I do in a case".

Group members' expectations of the group

Aside from the expectations of the supervision the group members need to have focus on themselves as a group. Raising this expectation early is a way to show how the supervision process will develop depending on how they behave as a group and towards each other. They participate in shaping the group climate and the group process. There is often a wish for an "open discussion", but it may have different meanings and therefore it's good if the group define what they mean:

"An open discussion means that we dare to express ourselves and our objections. Not get stuck by how I should express myself. Have permission to share what is weighing heavily on me. That it's a permissive environment, not judging".

Other expectations deal with how one should relate to each other. What do you want from each other? To reflect on how you want to relate to each other is important. Hearing how everyone is thinking stimulates group affinity and the group members are more likely to show their vulnerabilities and express expectations of each other.

"Accept each other for whom we are. We're different", "We pay attention and participate", "Listen actively to the person talking", "Respect for our own way of working", "That what is said in the room during supervision stays in the group",

"That we let go of prestige. Everyone is open about their difficulties", "That the group is open, down-to-earth. Not looking down on each other. We are people, after all. There is equality in the group regardless of our age or experience", "We can share what's funny, laugh about what's difficult, complement each other. We share our experiences and dare to show our vulnerabilities", "The group offers tips and advice. But sometimes I just want to share an experience and not be given tips and advice – not too fast", "Help and support each other. Dare to be ourselves", "I'm new in the role and want everyone to share their experiences".

There are some groups that are not open to each other and don't get on, and sometimes fail to keep focus on the client.

"We are cowards. We don't dare to ask questions at certain meetings. Who are the meetings for?", "In spite of being at the bottom we argue", "We lose sight of the children. It's sad".

I make a distinction between what one expects of the group and how one should be as a group. The question: "How do you want to be as a group?" is more of a challenge and straightforward. Some voices:

"Being a group that plants ideas and thoughts. Give space for these flowers to grow", "Find a calm approach. Use the energy that exists", "Being there for each other", "Focus on the work: What is the assignment?", "Focus more on creativity", "Disentangle what is our professional role", "Trusting each other. Hearing about one another's situation. Learn from one another", "Reflect on how we might get help from each other. What can we do together?".

Group member expectations of oneself

The supervision and group process and the way in which this develops does not only depend on the supervisor and the group but also on each group member. This is not necessarily obvious until the issue is raised. Then many say that they expect the same of themselves as of the group, i.e. to listen, to show respect, to participate and so on. As a supervisor I appreciate people talking about their openness and their willingness to come prepared to the supervision, having considered what they want to get from the supervision.

"I'm open and receptive to both criticism and advice. To feel secure in discussing the situation, that I'm actively participating", "Helping and contributing to my expertise", "I'm receptive and share my experiences. Supervision is a space where everything is acceptable", "To make the most of the supervision sessions",

"To learn. To feel I'm developing as much as much as possible", "To be myself", "To be positive", "To come a bit prepared. Contemplating what I want to get out of our meetings", "Participating. Give something of myself. Say what I think. Be straight and clear. Offering support", "To be honest, show respect for myself and others".

Expectations of the supervisor role

The role of leading the supervision is part of the supervision assignment. Supervisors may take different views of their role, just as group members have different expectations of the supervisor in that role. Certain expectations correspond to the role as such and the supervisor's own expectations. But there may also be expectations that are not part of the supervisor's role, or that the supervisor does not want to take on in the way the group would like. For my part I don't take the role of the one who presents solutions to any given problem or suggests what someone should do or how to behave. However, I'm ready to say what I might have done in the supervisee's situation. When group members raise some expectations of my role, I usually ask probing questions problematizing their request and sometimes assert that the issue is not part of my assignment, or proper to my role as supervisor. What do different group members say about their expectations of the supervisor's role?

"You are seeing things that I can't see. Subconscious notions I'm not aware of", "You have an open mind. Taking me seriously. You have an empathic attitude. You listen actively", "You ask: 'Is this what you want?' ", "It shouldn't lead to a conflict", "You guide us and make sure we're not overwhelmed by good advice", "You challenge us a bit", "You guide us", "You share your experiences", "You don't let things pass, as previous supervisors have done", "You control the process that the group doesn't take over", "You listen and are active. The person speaking has plenty of space", "You as supervisor bring matters to a good conclusion", "You make sure everyone expresses her view", "That you as supervisor know the group you are working with. You are seeing the group. What is it like? What support does it? Being guided. All groups are different",

"You get straight to the point. Directly. You ask in such a way that I have to put my thoughts into words", "I don't want to have my competence questioned or countered by prejudice. You as a supervisor can take criticism. Important to talk about the results", "You give new perspectives", "You are conducting the meeting", "You know what you're doing", "There is a structure", "You don't lecture us. You don't mess up our work, rather you contribute to the positive spirit we have", "You as supervisor don't talk about yourself. Not like our last supervisor who links his own experiences into what the person has experienced, whenever we are telling our case", "You dare to show how to manage and contain what is traumatic", "You are helping me to find new perspectives in a case. You contribute knowledge", "The supervisor is honest and has the capacity to notice and listen. It's hard when the supervisor doesn't understand".

The citations show that groups in general know what they expect of the supervisor. Even if the answer is "I don't know" in-depth questions help the individual to reflect. The ensuing dialogue usually clarifies what is requested of the supervision. The answers reveal what the group members are not satisfied with and what they do not want repeated. A group exemplifies how the previous supervisor behaved and doesn't want to see repeated by the next supervisor.

In the above citations there is an implicit expectation; the supervisor will both understand and accept what is being said without asking further questions to clarify what is meant. The supervisor is expected to maintain the structure, be able to deal what is difficult, know what the supervisees are doing and take them seriously, not lecture, and control the process.

Vague expectations of the supervisor's role will generate more in-depth questions already at the interview, for example, to understand what it means when the supervisor is asked to notice what the supervisee is not able to see himself. Such expectations need to be clarified – what should the supervisor be able to see? Understanding this correctly has implications for whether the supervisor can accept the task or not. Likewise, when the supervisor is expected to conduct and listen – what is supposed to be conducted and in what way? How would you know that the supervisor is listening? When someone expects challenges it's good to know what type of challenge one expects. Do we have the same connotation here – what is to be challenged, when and how?

When we discuss expectations of the supervisor's role my own view of supervision becomes more apparent, my supervision style and my attitude, including how I ask in-depth questions. The group learns more about me as a supervisor as I am acting in the interview, instead of just describing what I do.

2. Contact with manager or group leader

The management's role in supervision

Regarding supervision, the opinion and role of the management is often invisible. Some managers maintain contact with the supervisor at the start of the assignment and in agreeing on the contract but are otherwise not involved in the work of the supervisor in the supervision group, as regards content or process. Neither are there any explicitly stated expectations of the supervision by the managers.

Thylefors (2016) describes the role and task of the manager, which involves planning, organising, leading and controlling. What should be done is part of the work and assignment description and how such tasks should be performed is regulated by both formal and informal objectives. The manager should provide direction and state the goals of the mission, as well as to provide resources to achieve them, including to balance several interests. The manager is responsible for coordinating and allocating various items such as materials and human resources. The management should also set performance requirements, evaluate, and remedy problems. These functions are mutually dependent, according to Thylefors.

The role of manager includes the task of identifying and satisfying training needs of the co-workers. Supervision is one of several possible means to promote professional development of both the individual and the working group. Process supervision may be needed to stop a retrograde group development into previous and unwanted interactions. In the supervision new perspectives are opened, new opportunities to see one's role, the organisation and the work at hand can make a difference and facilitate change. A change such as new members or a changed attitude in the group may have impact on the individual group member's feelings and thoughts. Insights are reached and ensuing reflections may open new perspectives. Rogers (1976) argues that a changed perception of the self sooner or later unavoidably will show in behaviour. All "changes bring some form of confusion and more or less pain … when you learn something new about yourself and start to act based on this new self-knowledge, waves of consequences are generated that you can never fully predict" (s. 107).

The supervisor's contact and dialogue with the leader of the group and/or the manager is necessary. Supervision should not be an isolated activity, a matter only involving the supervisor and the supervisee. Process supervision affects individuals and the working group. Therefore, the supervisor must consider queries about the purpose and direction of the supervision also from the manager. The purpose and goals of the supervision can't be left to the supervisor and/or group members alone. The contact between the manager and the supervisor should have a clear purpose and be transparent to the members of the group. The manager should have as much insight in the supervision as necessary to judge whether it's in line with the contract, the assignment given to the supervisor and the expectations of the supervision; There should be no contradiction in what the supervisor, supervision group and manager are striving for, i.e. work with clients should be professional and of high quality as well as in line with the aims of the agency and its target group. The working group should have access to a space, a room for reflection and critical thinking, to find better solutions to their issues. Critical thinking demands time and maturity. To be able to reflect on the work together or alone, as well as in meetings with the target group. What is the response to specific meetings and what attitude should be adopted in response to certain situations?

In my supervision model I always establish contact with the group leader and/ or the manager. This contact is continuous during the entire assignment. The contact has a different purpose depending on where the group is in the supervision process and what we have agreed. I suggest contact with the manager at the start of the assignment, during the evaluation of the supervision once a year, or for specific questions raised during the supervision. The contacts focus the organisation, or the leadership. A contact with the manager is always first anchored in the supervision group and approved by the group members.

Contact prior to – and what can be raised in supervision

At the start of the assignment the supervisor and manager should be in contact – a contract should be drafted. At the time of the supervisor's interview with the group the supervisor should explain how she intends to be in touch with the manager. What should and will be communicated to the manager regarding content and the supervision process?

When a group has selected me as their supervisor, I want to meet the group manager. The reason is firstly to learn about his expectations of the supervision and of our contact. As a supervisor I need to know that I have the necessary competence and that I can meet the expectations the manager has of the supervision. Perhaps there are expectations I am unable to satisfy, or simply not ready to fulfil from my view of supervision, my ethical responsibility as supervisor and the confidence the group has granted me, all necessary for a successful supervision. For example, I never agree to certain areas being off limits for discussion in the supervision, such as the manager doesn't want the organisation or the leadership to be discussed. It's hard to deny the right to talk about such matters if affecting the supervisee's relationship with clients. On the other hand, I can always assure the manager that the supervision will not be turned into a forum for gossip and complaints about the manager or the agency.

In the long run process supervision doesn't focus management and organisation. Still, the supervisees might need to talk about this aspect when they try to figure out why they are unable to influence the organization or the leader. They may change their own attitude or way of dealing with problems by, for example, being more open, perceptive and participating, inviting communication from a Me-perspective taking responsibility for their own actions. In the supervision the supervisees gain an understanding and insight into what belongs in the personal sphere with its duties and responsibilities, and what type of influence you may have within the organisation or on the manager. You have a responsibility for the impact of your own attitude at the workplace. Rogers (1976) argues that open and honest communication of both thoughts and feelings, to raise issues and problems within the organisation of a concrete nature, achieves "real and perhaps irreversible change" (s. 97).

When the theme of the supervision on some occasions has been the manager and/or organisation I have suggested the group to bring this up with the manager. How this is done may vary depending on the contract agreement between the manager and the supervisor. Sometimes the supervision group speaks to the manager themselves. Or they might ask me to describe the issue at hand to the manager, or we agree to invite the manager to a supervision session and together explain what the group members want to communicate.

The manager's expectations of the supervision

I usually ask what the manager wants to know about the process and content of the supervision. As a rule, the manager has no opinion on the process and content of the supervision but wants to know if criticism is expressed regarding him, to be able do something about the situation.

Some managers' opinions on supervision

"Supervision strengthens the group as a group, in their professional roles and the relations between them. The supervision leads to better confidence within the group. There are possibilities for process and advice. It offers method and support at work."

"The supervision becomes a forum for good and constructive dialogue. The participants in the group should be straightforward towards one another. They can ask each other for help. Not just talk about the role as a mentor but also the role as colleagues."

"To talk about the manager's role if required. If there are critical views, it's fine to know to be able to improve. I expect the group to be active in the supervision and that everyone takes responsibility for the process."

"It's important that they may strengthen their professional role as social workers. They work alone so it's well if they can discuss how to be strong as a group. How they can help each other in difficult circumstances. Or see the possibility to do something together, me and them."

"In the supervision it's not just a matter of letting off steam by saying the boss is stupid. They should reflect on 'what's my part in this?' 'How could I develop?' 'How could I be good at my job?' The individuals should raise their own needs. They should know which clients they're working with, know what strategies to adopt when support is needed. We need to set limits even when there is low affectivity. If there is a fear of conflict in the group and the group members back down. They find it hard to see the entire picture. I expect them to be able to talk about this in the supervision."

"To gain an understanding of what their job is about. It's also important to look inside, see how their work influences the group and the clients with whom they are working."

"For me it's important to know if my staff working with trauma are suffering secondary traumatization."

The manager's role in evaluation of the supervision

At the interview the supervision group and supervisor agree that at least once a year the manager will attend an evaluation. Together it's decided on what will be disclosed to the manager. Before the manager arrives, an evaluation is made of the supervision. It works best when the manager beforehand knows how the meeting will be run and how the most important issues will be discussed. To have a dialogue within the group and give the manager an opportunity to ask whatever it is she wants to know, these are good starting points. On these occasions, questions may also be raised on forthcoming aims and expectations of the supervision, both those of the group and the manager.

Contact on specific issues raised in the supervision

If the group discussion has been focused on leadership or organisation, you often need to inform and discuss with the manager. It's not enough only to speak of it in the supervision. As I've already explained I usually reach an agreement at an early stage with the group members and the manager about what will happen if such a case arises. Some managers also include this provision in the contract. My experience is that one should not discuss issues of the organisation and leadership on more than two or three occasions during the supervision. It's preferable at the last session to discuss how information that emerges should be communicated to the leadership. There has perhaps been a discussion on the relationship with the manager, the way in which it impacts on group members, or on work with clients. No solution can be reached if the discussion is held only during the supervision. The manager should be involved and informed based on the agreement already in place, after discussing this in the group.

Writing a contract

The agreement is a written contract between the head manager of the agency and the supervisor. In the procurement documents different versions of possible contracts are described. Usually the manager drafts a contract, the supervisor approves and signs it after appropriate changes. A contract can be very short or contain all points agreed upon. I prefer the following to be included (examples of different contracts):

Formal details of the customer and service provider: mail and email address, company registration number, invoice address, telephone number.

Duration of contract, i.e. the scope and time period, including procedures in case of a cancellation or discontinuation.

The aim of the supervision/assignment (short description). An example: "Supervision of staff doing social work for children. The supervision is providing an opportunity to deal with the processes affecting the staff in their work. In addition, giving the staff an opportunity to reflect on and deepen the work with the target group." Or it might just state: "Process supervision". Or as in another contract: "Assignment 2018 regarding external/process supervision: Child and youth work in SDF ... is driven consciously by holistic thinking from a client perspective – the supervisor is responsible for this perspective to inform the supervision. The aim of *'Children and Youths'* is to approach the client from a distinct child-, gender-, and equality perspective – the supervisor is responsible for this perspective to inform the supervision. Reflection/training to make optimal use of each other in internal/external cooperation and in one's individual process. Awareness of how one is affected by parallel processes and projections. One's own therapeutic role."

Rules of participation and attendance for group members (what is specified, i.e. the supervision is a compulsory undertaking for all; when are participants allowed to take leave of absence?). For example: "Attendance is compulsory. The staff will arrive on time and are responsible for their active participation in the supervision."

Structure of feedback to the manager (what is to be communicated, when, by whom and how). For example: "The supervisor provides feedback to the responsible manager once per term. Additional feedback may be given when necessary." Another example: "To provide feedback to the principal of the assignment if the focus of the supervision repeatedly refers to organisational or other issues related to the working environment, issues which can only be resolved between the employer and employee."

Evaluation and date when the manager should be in attendance. For example: "The principal of the assignment will attend the final supervision session in the contract period. The supervisor and supervision group will then provide feedback on the content of the supervision during this period." Or: "In consultation with the group and NN an evaluation will be provided focusing on: Has the supervision been useful, have the goals of the supervision been fulfilled? Does the supervision contribute to professional development? How to proceed? What goals should be in focus?"

Contact person (most often the supervisor and the group agree on a contact person).

The premises, where are the premises to be and who will book it. (It's not always the supervisor who has access to premises. In such a case the group books the premises and the fee is lowered by the corresponding amount).

Fee and remuneration. (This is usually agreed during the contract negotiation, if there is one. Otherwise the manager and the supervisor decide on the price)

Content of the invoice. (Along with the necessary documentation of names, business registration numbers, address, bank or postal giro, the precise number of hours and dates of the supervision, the price and VAT, are stipulated. Sometimes the manager wants to include the number of participants with names).

Certificate. (After the completion of the supervision each participant in the supervision is to receive a certificate stipulating the period and hours of attendance of the supervision. The supervisor briefly describes the contents of the supervision).

Cancellation/extension. (Here the procedure is stated in case of cancellation or extension of the contract).

Terms of payment. (Usually it's a month).

Signatures and dates.

3. The supervision begins

Introductory lecture on unconscious processes

In the beginning of the supervision assignment I give a lecture on unconscious processes – see below – and give a short explanation of my supervision model and how I use these concepts during sessions. In my experience, a theoretical outline at the start of the supervision leads to a better understanding of the processes that arise and reinforces trust in the working method. In the dialogue between the supervisee and myself, the supervisee attains what processes are activated within herself, what these may depend on and what they recall.

It's up to the supervisor to define the difference between supervision and therapy, a distinction implying that the supervisee must not reveal more about herself than required to understand the interaction and process between herself and the client and/or herself and the supervisor. The supervisor does not ask questions regarding private life and "protects" the supervisee, so she does not reveal more than necessary.

The academic literature often describes unconscious processes as exposed in a psychotherapeutic relationship. In my experience they also often show in other professional relationships, even when no psychotherapeutic relation is at hand. As the client/patient finds himself in a position of dependency, the unequal relationship may prompt feelings of vulnerability in relation to the professional. It may develop in relation, for example, to a social worker who is in a position of power in her role and assignment. She might judge and define the client's financial situation, comment on lifestyle, "demand" changes and emphasise consequences in case such changes do not occur. This power and control function to "direct and decide" the client's way of life and behaviour is legally defined. The client may experience this as a child-parent relationship or as a power relationship, confirming a feeling of inferiority. Knowledge of unconscious processes and what shapes them helps the professional to relate to the client in a constructive and curative manner, instead of dismissing the client's reactions as if the client is considered not motivated to change, or hard to reach.

The following concepts are introduced to the supervision group at the start of a supervision assignment: *projection, induction, resonance, transference and countertransference, projective identification, and parallel processes.*

Projection

Projection is a joint term for psychological mechanisms which entail thoughts, feelings, impulses and/or structures within oneself being transferred to someone else, or to something in one's surrounding. Something undesirable within oneself is attributed to someone else, something to be suppressed, such as anxiety-inducing or unacceptable impulses and qualities. In this way, what is projected is experienced as characteristic of the other person. Projection is used as a defence mechanism by those who strive to rid themselves of what causes pain and distress and prompts feelings of distaste. It is a tendency to blame others for one's own failings. One is distrustful and prejudiced towards other people, especially if they are strangers, or different in some essential way from oneself. A projection does not require any relationship between the person projecting and the one being attributed a projection. However, there are situations when the subject of a projection is affected by the attitudes and actions of the other one.

Induction

Induction or charging is described by Belin (1993) as feelings raised by the active emotional influence of another. One is "charged" by what is induced. An influence like induction may only arise when there is a relation between two persons. As a therapist one is drawn into a strong force field in the relation to the client. This is especially true when working with psychotic patients or individuals with early disturbed relationships. Belin (1993) argues that the feelings with which the therapist is charged have nothing to do with herself. When the patients themselves are incapable of dealing with their own charged emotions they seek "supportive carriers" for their inner emotional chaos "by inducing (charging) different feelings and experiences in the caretakers. This occurs through open, dramatic as well as subtle activities" (s. 36). For the client the personal and vital relationship is necessary to the functioning of the emotional process. Belin argues that we are affected by various emotional force fields. Some people fill us with high spirits and energy, while others make us feel tired, empty, dead. This influence has an impact on us and on the relationship to the other with whom we have such a response. It can be all too easy to ascribe one's feelings to someone else and therefore good self-knowledge is necessary to recognise the origins of such feelings.

Currently we speak of mirror neurons, that we all have and through which we might feel what others are feeling.

Resonance

Resonance arises in human interaction when a person's feelings and moods connect to feelings and moods already present in another one. It may help the therapist to identify with or feel empathy for the individual she is talking to. The resonance may however stimulate almost unbearable feelings if it touches areas within the therapist that are conflictual, subconscious and/or unprocessed. This may harm the interaction as the arising emotions are hard to deal with. Resonance develops because of the therapist's receptivity (Belin, 1993).

Transference

Transference (Evang, 1991) is an emotional response of the client in relation to the therapist. Such responses originate in the client's earlier experiences and interpersonal relationships. Emotional responses are transferred from the past to the present. For example, the client may accuse the therapist of not listening, of not being pedagogic, of not liking him or wishing him well, of not being helpful and so on. These accusations do not necessarily depend on the actual behaviour and personality of the therapist, rather they may originate in earlier experiences of the client in relation to significant individuals. The therapist should understand these mechanisms to avoid feeling personally offended and unfairly treated, or to start arguing with the client.

Countertransference

Countertransference may be described as an instrument by which the therapist can gain a deeper understanding of the client. Igra (1988) defines countertransference as all those feelings, fantasies and activities evoked in the therapist by the interaction with the client's personality. It is about the inner reactions of the professional – covering processes that are a mixture of past and present, reality and fantasy, outside and inside, conscious and subconscious. The professional recognises an actual quality in the client and its significance in terms of her own personal history and characteristic defence. Her personal history has an impact as she may subconsciously, for example, perceive the client as her lying father because the client is behaving like a lying person. The problematic side of countertransference arises if the professional then starts to treat her client as if he was her father. Igra argues that the professional in countertransference may enter a neurotic interaction with the client in which earlier anxieties and psychological defences are triggered in the professional. In such a case the healthy interest in the client is lost and the situation becomes part of a personal process, rather than using one's subjective response to advance an understanding of the client's inner state and the client's motives for being untruthful.

According to Tähkä (1987) a countertransference always tends to complicate treatment as it may cause the therapist to entirely misunderstand the client or interpret the client's problem in a way that does not correspond to reality. Negative countertransference may cause the therapist to lose sympathy for the client. Typical types of countertransference according to Tähkä are statements like the client is the one with a problem, or the client is evil and manipulative. Such conclusions prevent the professional from seeing the client as a person with serious problems, someone who is frightened and in need of treatment.

Diagnostic countertransference is a concept used among others by Casement (1986) to describe the way in which the therapist through countertransference can access feelings the client may have in interplay with others. In the therapeutic relationship similar interactions and emotional responses may arise as those existing in the client's relation to his environment.

Complementary reactions are a type of countertransference shaped in relation to the client. It refers to the professional's constructive reactions when responding to a client's need to be understood and cared for in a certain way. For example, feelings of empathy and recognition are evoked in the professional by the vulnerable child hidden within the adult person. In certain situations, it becomes natural to act in a complementary way in relation to the client's incapacity by offering, for example, protection, comfort, or guidance.

Projective identification

Projective identification functions, according to Belin (1993), as:
- *a defence* to create distance to undesirable aspects and feelings in oneself
- a *means to communicate* to arouse feelings in others to be understood
- a *means of relating* to someone who is significant

Projective identification takes place in three phases. These should be included to be able to talk about projective identification as communication, according to Ogden (1987). In phase one, the client has unconscious fantasies about getting rid of something within oneself, such as feelings of being worthless or alienated, fear, uneasiness, sadness, or anger. To be freed from emotions, an interpersonal interaction is needed, which is phase two. In the interplay, the client behavior makes the professional respond in a way corresponding to the projective imagination. In a treatment situation, for example, the professional, after the unconscious communication with the client, can be afflicted by feelings of uncertainty, worthlessness, anger, sadness, or fear while the client is experiencing a kind of relief. How the professional deals with the emotions he has by induction „taken in" from the client becomes crucial for phase three in the projective identification process. In this phase the projected will again be internalized. The professional's experience is like what the client experienced in phase one. Only if the professional can cope with the emotions in a different way than the client, a processing of the projected may occur. The client's ability to process the undesirable lies in identifying with the professional and his way of keeping and dealing with what has been uncovered. The intention is that the client takes back a processed and digested projection, which he tried to get rid of. The reinternalization consists of both the projected and the way in which the projected has been processed.

If the reader wants to look more into the supervisor's interventions and how supervisors in different cases concretely work with these concepts, I refer to the book Supervision – The Therapist's Creative room (Cajvert, 2013).

Parallel processes

Parallel processes are problems, virtual blockings, patterns, solutions, and developments that arise in two simultaneous ongoing relationships: the relationship of the professional – client and the relationship of the supervisor – the professional. How the professional describes the client's problem may also express the professionals , own problem in the supervision process. Or the supervisor's difficulty and problem in understanding the supervisee may be the expression of parallel processes, the supervisor's problem to understand his client. The supervision thus replicates problems the supervisee has with the client. The supervisee „becomes" in the supervision situation to some extent „his client". Belin (1993) argues that in the discovery of parallel processes there is a chance for the professional and supervisor to find ways to move forward in a locked situation. It is more difficult to work with parallel processes in groups, and of course with those professionals who have no interest and/or theoretical basis for these processes or do not have the ability to perceive them.

The supervisor is a part of these processes and therefore it is important that he can recognize feelings that arise in the supervision process and identify their origins in the same way that the supervisee gets help to identify her emotions in the relationship to the client.

4. The supervision session

Stages of the session

There are many ways to start and to organise a supervision session. How the supervisor introduces the content and how the process develops depends on the supervisor's theoretical background and specific supervision style. Here I will introduce a model I have developed over many years, and almost always use. It suits my personal style and is aimed at helping the supervisees to become active and allow the one in focus to get an answer to his supervision question.

This model of the supervision session is briefly presented during the first interview. A group that chooses the supervisor, implicitly mandates her to use her model. This can be a problem when not everyone in the group attended the interview or when new members join the group. The supervisor's presentation must then be repeated. To avoid having everyone listening once more to the presentation the supervisor may ask first-time attendees to arrive an hour before the others. This has been shown to work well. My model of supervision has a clear outline and structure as well as flexibility within these limits. The supervisor follows a main thread and encourages the group members to participate in the supervision. She is active and has a responsibility to maintain the structure, to get an answer to the supervision question of the supervisee in focus, and to ensure the group process does not turn into a general discussion or a chat. The role and responsibility of the supervisor include continuous listening to everyone and as the process develops setting up new mini contracts.

The starting point is: What does the supervisee want to focus on in his supervision question? In what way should the group members and supervisor be active to resolve the question? How the process develops depends on the level of trust and alliance created between the group and the supervisor. A working alliance, mandate and trust are all necessary for the outcome of the method. The supervision session has different stages, and each stage has a purpose in terms of what needs to be done, how and why. The stages are divided as follows:
- Opening stage
- Feedback and choice of supervision question
- Formulating a supervision question
- The supervision process

- Bridging the supervision question and the work context
- Feedback on the supervision session

Opening

The supervision session may start by the supervisor using a variety of techniques helping the group participants to *"settle in the supervision room"*. The purpose is to create an atmosphere conducive to thoughts, feelings, and reflection.

The opening of the session may involve the use of cards, images or asking a simple question: "Where are you right now?" It's an open question and everyone may start with himself or herself and what one wishes to share, relate to, or reflect over. It may be something from work, something personal or private. The supervisor doesn't control the content. Anything should be permissible to share. Pictures help everyone to open one's mind and start associating freely. Starting like this also makes a statement: "In this room we're doing something different. The supervision begins now". Work and everyday life is left behind, and we can focus our attention on the supervision here and now. This may help the supervisees to sharpen their mental presence and it may also have a relaxing effect.

The materials the supervisor may use in the opening stage are described in greater detail in part 5.

Feedback and choice of supervision question

After the *opening* stage the supervisor makes a note of who are present and asks if anyone in the group knows why someone is absent. This information is intended only for the supervisor and is part of the basis for the certificate group members get after completed supervision, as agreed in the contract.

Feedback on the previous supervision session

The supervisor might want to know if group members want to share anything positive or negative from the previous session. The question allows the group members to reflect on something they have learned and have been of use to them. Feedback is important to the supervisor who learns what has functioned well, but also if anyone has been misunderstood or if the supervisor has failed to help a group member with his supervision question. If the group after a supervision session talk amongst themselves about a possible discontent with the session, the supervisor should get to know about it. To put this question at the start of each session also gives an opportunity and an invitation to be open about someone in the group, or perhaps the entire group, having a less positive experience of the latest session. This gives the supervisor a chance to reflect on and fix any possible misunderstanding. It's a chance for all to learn from experience – both the group members and the supervisor. The supervisor's attitude should be that she takes any discontent seriously and is prepared to try to do something about it. It's important not to become defensive or place the blame on someone. How the supervisor is dealing with the discontent of group members may offer a model for them to deal with discontent occurring among their clients.

Who has brought a supervision question

Who has brought a supervision question or an issue you wish to raise? This question is open and put to each participant. It's enough if each one gives a yes or no answer to this question. The supervisor gains an idea of how many who wish to be in focus. If more than two participants answer Yes, they wish to raise something, the supervisor discusses with the group how to prioritise. All are then asked to briefly describe their question or issue, what they wish to gain from the supervision and how urgent the problem is. This makes it easy to prioritise, plan and allocate available time. During a supervision session of three hours I can complete two supervision processes, or three supervision questions if the process is more limited in scope. With three questions the supervision becomes more of a consultation. It's a mutual undertaking to be responsible for who will have the opportunity to raise their issue. It's not unusual for several in the group to want to raise a shared issue, or a theme which concerns some members or the entire group.

When no one has any issue to raise

It happens in nearly every group that the participants at some point arrive at the supervision without anyone having an issue to raise. How should the supervisor respond? She may ask the supervision group how they want to use the time of the session. That question usually prompts someone to raise an issue, and it's not unusual for several of the members to "take on the challenge" in such a situation. However, if in the end no one in the group has any question to raise, the supervisor may suggest a previously raised topic not yet sufficiently discussed.

The supervisor may have prepared some exercises which activate the group and the group process. If no one repeatedly is bringing along an issue on several occasions the supervisor should put this to the group and ask the members to reflect: "Why do you not have any questions to raise?" Together the supervisor and the group will reach a solution for and an idea about how to move the supervision forward. A new contract will then be created on how to proceed in the case of no one having any issues to raise and on how the supervisor must then respond. Often, this may start the supervision anew.

Formulate a supervision question

Defining the supervision question is the basis for maintaining focus on what the supervisee wishes to raise and get support for. For other group members and the supervisor it is also a question of knowing how to listen and what further information is required to understand the question and be able to share reflections and thoughts. The supervision question does not have to be ready and prepared in advance of the supervision, rather the supervisor may help defining the issue. Only when the supervision question is ready the supervision process will continue. I always write the supervision question on the board, along with how the supervisee wishes to make use of the group.

Sometimes the supervisee will bring along a supervision question but requires help to frame it in the session. He knows what he is wrestling with, what the problem is, but need help expressing his question. Sometimes he first wishes to describe the issue, then to frame the supervision question. This takes place through dialogue and by agreeing a mini contract with the supervisor. Based on a variety of supervision settings in different professional groups, here are three different examples of how to approach the supervision question:
1. The supervisee has a supervision question ready.
2. The supervisee needs help to formulate his supervision question.
3. The supervisee wants first to describe a problem and based on this to arrive at a supervision question.

The supervisee has a question ready

Group members sooner or later get used to have their supervision question formulated before the session. They know what they want to address.

The supervision question may relate to anything from not knowing how to approach a child, a parent, or a colleague, to wanting to understand certain feelings evolving when meeting a specific client. It may also relate to how it is at work, amongst colleagues or in relation to the manager.

When the supervisor asks the question: "What is your supervision question?", perhaps the question needs to be clarified and it may take a while before it makes sense to the supervisee.

Here are some examples of questions that may be used when various themes are in focus within different activities. These questions may deal with dialogue, approach, or attitudes, but also how one is affected emotionally by the work.

When the dialogue is in focus:
- What should I do to be distinct in my next communication with the client?
- I am going to talking to children. What is most important to think about? What may I raise?
- How can I deal with youths after a rejected visa? How to deal with other youths involved?
- What should I do to be more distinct?

When the approach and attitude is in focus:
- How should I address a child, who asks so many questions?
- How should I approach a father who affects me strongly when we talk? I don't want any contact with him.
- How to approach an ambivalent father?
- How do I move on? I am so tired of talking to them.
- The family can't cooperate. I want to help the kid, but I don't know how.
- How should we cooperate and not blaming the guys before we know what happened?
- How do we set limits for colleagues and other professionals?
- What is important to communicate when roles are unclear?
- How to protect yourself without shutting off your emotions?

When the supervisee is affected by his work and doesn't know what to do the supervision question may be framed as follows:

- Should I continue to participate in a task when I can't support the decision?
- How do unclear rules affect the group? What does this do to us as individuals and as a group?
- How should I distance my thoughts and feelings from the problems facing the youths and not bring my concerns back home? I want tools, ideas, and suggestions.
- I want to help the kid but don't know how.
- Why do I feel like this? Why am I affected negatively by the client?
- Want help to deal with my feelings. Many feelings: insecurity, stress, sole responsibility.
- Frustrated by not knowing what to do.
- Who should decide what in my case? Is there a power struggle? How to settle this dilemma?

The supervisee needs help to formulate a question

It's not unusual that you want to raise an issue but lack a distinct supervision question and need help to frame it. Through a dialogue, most often between the supervisor and the individual in focus, he gets help in formulating his supervision question. A brief explanation of the issue may be necessary, about the process or about the feelings and reactions towards the client, to extract a supervision question.

When new to the supervision group, the workplace or to this supervision model, it may be difficult right from the start to formulate your supervision question. You might need help to see what you want. Perhaps the group and the supervisor need to know more about the background to the situation where the feeling arose to frame the supervision question. After describing the feelings, thoughts, and the situation in general the following types of supervision questions may be formulated, not unlike the questions you would frame when you already know what to focus:

- How to address the client and adopt an adequate attitude?
- How to approach the client without telling him like "pull yourself together"?
- How to approach the mother justifying a decision to revoke custody?
- How to approach youths who don't follow rules?

- I have two contradictory ideas about the client and is caught in both while talking to him. How should I avoid doing this?
- Transfer of custody: we have different thoughts on this. How to raise the issue without hurting anyone?
- Desperate situation when youths are sent to death. How should I relate to my work when I am a part of the Swedish community?
- Find an approach when I see deceit by the community.
- I don't think I'm doing enough. I should do more.

Just describe a problem and then frame a question

Often, the supervisee wants to describe the problem before the supervision question is framed. Here are some examples.

The supervisee just wants to describe a problem and the process involved. He wants to tell loudly and thus gain some relief. Sometimes he is not even interested in hearing the thoughts and ideas of the group or the supervisor, the point is simply to tell and that's okay. Often, he himself will arrive at something he finds helpful or develops an idea on how to move on.

The supervisee might want to describe a certain situation and hear how the group would respond in a similar situation or wants to receive tips and advice on how to move on. It may also be a matter of wanting confirmation that you did the right thing. This could also be a supervision question, but the wish is to relate the whole chain of events in one's own words.

There are situations in which you doubt if a question is relevant to the supervision and in that case, you want to explain before any supervision question is formulated. There may also be some doubts as to whether the question is a matter of method or if it is a question to be raised in process supervision.

It may be difficult to speak of your own dilemmas and thoughts, especially if it relates to a colleague, your relation to the manager or something you have experienced at work. You may be uncertain whether this belongs in the supervision.

In such circumstances the supervisor could request a short presentation of what the supervisee wants to achieve by relating the situation. How did the incident influence his professional work? What help does he want to handle the concrete situation?

Other examples may be the need to talk about certain "endless issues" and how to relate to such recurring issues.

Some questions expressed as short notes:
- I can't generate any energy at work.
- I'm a happy person but in this job, I start fretting and snap at people. I want my own image of how I am to fit better.
- What sort of group are we? How do we behave towards one another?
- Stress and frustration of running out of time. Lacking certain knowledge.
- Don't have any contact with the manager.
- Health, how is it affected by work?
- Feeling insufficient. How to cope?
- Don't want to take part in this work and being cynical about reality.
- Need energy.
- State of health and stress.
- Help in dealing with emotions.
- To be acknowledged for what I do.
- Lack appreciation from the manager for my daily work.

These supervision questions are not easy to formulate without lengthy explanations and stories. You need time to bring up the dilemmas, needs, thoughts and feelings around the issues you are wrestling and want to focus

The supervision process

This stage of supervision process is the essence of the supervision and will take the longest time. The stage is characterised by pauses and process. Here creativity develops, an area of play where thoughts and reflections may prosper and deepen the process.

When the supervision question and how the group should be used are decided, a process of questions, dialogue and collection of materials begins. The whole group problematizes, all group members participate and may ask questions. There is room for using images and other creative techniques to trigger the discussion. The supervisee selects the form, but the supervisor may also make suggestions.

The supervisor helps to maintain a common thread by keeping the group members at the topic and making sure that questions are related to the task set by the supervisee. This makes everyone active in the supervision process. There is no room for an appraisal nor questioning of other members comments. One may ask questions that deepen the thoughts of the other. In this stage the story is unravelled. The narrative takes shape and becomes distinct. If there was a dilemma it will be revealed. What he has tried and failed or succeeded to accomplish is shown. The supervisee's thoughts, feelings and difficulties and his assignment are elucidated from several perspectives. This process culminates in the activity of the whole group according to what the supervisee wanted the group to contribute and do. What has been unravelled is then jointly analysed, coupled to theory and considered from different perspectives. The supervisee in focus should at the end of this process and the chosen method of reflection and participation of the other members have an answer to his supervision question.

During the process the supervisor supports the supervisee to clarify the following:

- What is your task in this specific job? Focus the task.
- What *do* you *have to* do? Focus what you *must* do. For example, what must be done according to the assignment, the task, the law, goals of the organization etc.
- What *can* you do? Focus is on what is possible based on the task at hand, the resources of the organization and its scope. But also considering the competence of the supervisee and the needs of the client and his readiness of accepting help. Who does the supervisee need to contact to carry out the task?
- What do you *want* to do? Focus is on what the supervisee wants to do. When he has formulated what he wants to do, the supervisor should again emphasise: is it within the framework of your task? Is it in line with the client's needs and wishes? Do you have the competence to do what you want to do? In that case what tools do you need? Who do you need to talk to before you act?

By clarifying to himself what needs to be done, what can be done and what he want to do, the supervisee may distinguish what is included in the task and raise his awareness of whether this is in line with the expectations of the client, or whether he himself has an idea of what would be the best for the client in the present situation. The supervisor also is tasked to help the supervisee not to be burdened by doing what is not within the scope of the task, his competence, or the expectations of the client.

Bridge to the work context

What does the supervisee want to do with what he has "got" from the supervision? How is this going to work? The supervisee and the supervisor make a summary together and sometimes suggested solutions are written on the board. In what order should the chosen approaches be used, what needs to be done, when and with whom to achieve the best solution to the supervision question. At this stage the supervisor may contribute a brief theoretical explanation or introduce a model which may be applicable in some way. The supervisee should always feel comfortable in using what is being suggested. It is always the supervisee who has "the last word" on what might be useful to him.

It is the supervisee in dialogue with the supervisor who builds a bridge between the supervision process and his work context, within the limits of what is possible at his work, his own capacity and the client's needs and problems.

Review of the supervision session and feedback

After each addressed supervision question, the supervisor asks what has worked and what has been useful, also what each participant will take away from the supervision. Everyone makes a brief comment and after a short break the next supervision question is posed.

Feedback is useful for the supervisor and group members to consider doing something differently, if necessary, to understand and practise what works; feedback is conducive to professional development. The supervisor learns how methods used were beneficial to each participant.

Supervision is a lonely job and it's important for the supervisor to get feedback from the supervisees. Group members practise their ability in giving but also in receiving feedback. This makes them more confident in applying what they have learned in their professional work with clients.

5. Tools and approaches in supervision

The importance of reflection

Supervision is a forum for reflection and thinking about your work and professional role together with other professionals. Reflection is important for understanding your own actions, yourself, and the person to whom you are talking. When the supervisee describes his client, it is his idea of the client and the client's problems that is discussed and not that of the client. The client is not present, and the supervisee's description is trusted. In the supervision, space is created for the supervisee to reflect on:

- his attitude and idea about the client and the client's problems
- the feelings, responses and processes that arise when meeting the client
- his theoretical knowledge, how he uses it and what impact it has on the therapeutic relationship
- his view of man, his values, and attitudes important for a professional approach in meeting the client.

When a question is formulated, and a dilemma or problem is in focus the supervisee is not the only one reflecting. The entire group and the supervisor contribute with reflections as desired. They broaden the perspective, and help seeing the problem from a variety of theoretical approaches – their thoughts are simply shared on the topic raised. Professional communication requires reflection. Regardless of the method the supervisor is applying all are based on an element of reflection. Bie (2012) writes that reflection sometimes entails observing yourself and your own reactions. It's a communication about actions and experiences. Reflection is a process, it's more than thinking and more than talking. It's a tool for a systematic and conscious learning; you observe yourself from the outside.

Reflection is necessary to develop theoretical and practical knowledge and a professional identity. You use reflection as a strategy for active learning. It's a conscious seeking to understand something, to gain another perspective on yourself, to look upon yourself with new eyes and gain another understanding of yourself and your actions. The focus may be on experiences, thoughts and feelings, understanding and knowledge, how you relate to the world and to other professionals, your attitude, ability to assess and your perspectives. It's about trying to grasp the very meaning of what you are reflecting upon. Through reflection you learn to sort knowledge and its use, to develop your critical thinking and becoming aware of what knowledge you already have, and what should be developed and on what you should focus. You gain an understanding of how to communicate and an insight into the significance of emotions in work and in collaboration with colleagues and others. Reflection creates learning tools for how to learn. The result of reflection might be that you change your course of action and understanding of the situation reflected upon. Reflection helps when deciding and improves the ability to practise and integrate theoretical knowledge and practical skills. A prerequisite for reflection is a readiness to start a process where you directly observe your own experiences (Bie, 2012).

Tools to help reflecting on a supervision question

To achieve a dynamic and inspiring supervision the supervisor usually applies a variety of methods and working materials. When and how the various methods are used depends on the aim of using a specific method or work materials. The materials are in most cases cards, images, taped dolls, and model figures, such as Playmobil. The method could be a role play – "if you were this person", "if this was my client", a reflecting team listening to a range of voices and ideas, silent positioning and so forth.

Mainly, I ask the supervisee how he wants to use the group and what method he would like to use. If the group is not familiar with the method, I give a brief description. Sometimes I may suggest a method or working materials right from the start, based on the supervision question.

Here I will briefly describe the content of some of these methods and when the supervisor might use them. Before selecting a method, the supervisor, and the supervisee, might consider:

- What is the supervision question?
- Who should be in focus?
- Why should the method be used?
- Is it relevant to the current situation?
- How safe is the group: how long have they been in supervision, how well do they know each other?
- Could the supervisee and group be challenged and to what degree?
- At what stage of development is the supervisee in focus and the supervision group as a group?

- Who are their clients – will they benefit from this method?
- What is the level of competence of the supervisee?

Even if all this is important and the supervisor tries considering all these matters, she sometimes misses and uses a method not suitable for the group, and which the group does not see any use for either for themselves or their clients.

The supervisor should try to be perceptive to which method that might be suitable and give clear instructions. Sometimes, when a method is new to me, I have also been uncertain and hence provided inadequate instructions.

I try to use methods I am comfortable with and use those I have already tried myself in various courses and workshops. When I use a deck of cards there are instructions that come with the various decks, but I also tend to find my own way of working with the cards. In the text below I will, rather than describing different cards, cite what groups have said about them. The citations from these individuals also express their feelings and describe what they have gained personally from the use of the cards.

Using pictures and cards

I've realised that different cards and pictures may have a both stimulating and inhibiting effect when used in supervision. The supervisee might feel obliged to say something about the cards, but momentarily lacks imagination or anything to share, compared to what others have said, etcetera. It may be that he does not want to reveal too much. Therefore, it should be voluntary whether one takes part. But a voluntary element in a mutual activity is not without its problems. If one group member regularly chooses not to participate it creates an imbalance in the group. It may also be difficult to become part of the group if from the start one chooses not to participate. It's the task of the supervisor to create a dialogue and on a meta-level discuss the situation that arises. It's important not "name and shame" any individual, not to make a judgement or criticise, to avoid even more of a deadlock instead of an opening. Clients may also deadlock during treatment, finding it hard to express themselves, to explain or share information with the therapist. When similar situations occur in supervision everyone can learn, and the supervisor can be a model for how such conditions may be resolved.

To freely associate about pictures shown on a drawn card may also be revealing. More is revealed about yourself than was intended or desired. Your values are exposed, your view of the client or the client's problems. It may be something you were not ready to share with the group. You may be surprised about what it says of your view of man, your judgement or desire to punish the client or those with whom you are working. If this happens it's important that the person concerned feels safe, both within the group and in relation to the supervisor. But sometimes the method can be challenging and if the group members furthermore do not know one another they may choose to cancel the supervision assignment.

The cards I usually use are: pictures of various chairs; the Saga deck; Feelings and needs; OH-cards using both words and images; Persona card deck of different faces; SAGOLEK IKEA; Habitat; Emotive card figures; More than one story – to name a few.

Pictures and cards to start

The supervisor can start off the supervision session with a picture card that group members select from the deck and then freely talk about. Each one may associate to his professional or private life, or wherever he now finds himself. If the supervisor wants to vary the pictures, she can make a note of what type of card she has been using and use different ones each time.

Using cards to start off the supervision session should take a maximum of 15 minutes in a group of six. It's not unusual that someone reveals something of which the group had not previously been aware. It may be personal and sometimes private. Group members form a closer bond and gain a greater understanding of each other's qualities and experiences. I usually don't note down any personal information revealed by what was told from the cards. Sometimes I will make a note on whether someone is talking about her work or the group process.

Here are some examples of what supervisees have said about cards when used to start the supervision:

"Good start, it gets us on the way", "Unexpected questions", "Good to listen to the others", "Everyone in the group is interested", "Good to start with the cards. It gets the supervision going. The supervision enters the room", "Makes everyone visible", "Cards used at the start of the supervision functions as a gate into the supervision situation, now you can get going. Good start", "I stop thinking about work, what I've done and what has not been completed", "You must think – reflect, now we're in the supervision", "You share something personal and that is a positive process for the group. Good introduction to get your emotions going", "It's pleasant to start off with the cards. Positive things and memories come up",

"Sets the emotional level for the day", "Everyone shares something of themselves", "We land a little. Can take the stress out of the day. Creates a mood of presence. Good start", "The day begins in harmony. Becomes more relaxed", "Cards mean that one is forced to answer, to say something. Quickly get in the mood for the supervision", "I like cards as it helps us to get to know one another. See what people are thinking. Cards strengthens us as a team. Everyone is focused on the here and now. Forced to focus. To reflect".

"Cards provide a distinct start; you get in the mood. Now it's time for process supervision. Exciting to listen to the others. You open yourself up for something. For communication, sharing about yourself.

"Sometimes I want to talk about something and then I hope you've brought along the cards. Then I get the chance to raise it. Opens a door that is shut. Good to talk about one's emotions", "Get disappointed if there are no cards. I like games", "Cards are sometimes difficult to connect with anything", "It's harder when it's just a picture. For me it's better when there are words".

There are, however, occasions when I write down what is said, for example when I use different chairs and ask: "Which chair are you on right now?" and everyone selects a chair. Often it has to do with work and how they are feeling at that moment. I take notes at this point because which chair they're on has to do with their situation at work. The cards sometimes stir up strong emotions and then we slow down and talk about it.

Here follow some examples of what group members might mention when the task is to say something about the chosen chair. They show their chair to everyone:

"The chair is uncomfortable. Straight back. The atmosphere has changed at work. From friendly to formal. Boring to be so stiff. The framework is clearer but more formal power is used. It becomes stiff and I lean against these inflexible rules." Or: "That chair looks boring. Modest but not comfortable. I feel no energy at work. It feels boring. Sad to return home not having energy for anything."

"Sit on a chair, the wheels are spinning. It's better at work now. Feels good. The work has not really changed. Start to roll forward and I feel I'm becoming part of the new group. Important not to get stuck and drawn into what is bad."

"I should sit on my own chair and not get too involved as I usually do. I tend to always come up with new ideas."

"I don't sit comfortably in this chair which I am slipping out of – can't stay in my seat. At work I don't get any support from my manager. Nobody asks how it's going. There's a lot of worry among the guys. I'm also worried. Upset. Failing trust. Who can we trust? I'm not safe in my chair."

"It's an active chair. I'm always on the go. I can sit on the chair to recuperate. Good things have happened in life despite crises. I choose the good moments. Happy with my existence."

"I feel calmer. Started to accept what I can't change. I have no influence over what is happening."

"Sitting comfortably in the chair right now. Can fold it when it's not needed any more."

"Sitting steadily on this chair. I feel stable right now. I feel appreciated. Find strength in myself. I can manage. At ease at work. I'm surrounded by great colleagues. I'm appreciated. I enjoy my leisure time. Solve a lot of problems. Nothing can stop me."

"The seat is comfortable. It's a stable chair. At work everything is now just right. Going abroad to bathe. I'm satisfied and life feels comfortable. Life is just right."

"My chair is balancing on an edge. Sometimes it's tough – trying to keep my balance and not fall off the chair. Full-time job, small kids, should try to get out to enjoy myself."

"It's a smooth ride. Everything is in order but a little boring. Need to travel. I like it here. Want something more, want something to look forward to."

"Happy, things are easy at work. Have a stable footing. Still a little bit wobbly."

When a group express themselves as in the above citations – "it is comfortable now" – I might ask: "What has made you end up where you are?" Some answers I get:

"At work things are going well, among us colleagues", "Our group is very stable right now", "We have a reasonable workload in terms of cases", "Good support from the management and the head of the organisation", "We all help one another", "We accept our differences. We help each other. In our group nothing is left unresolved. We're a good agency".

In my experience I can clearly see when a group is at ease with one another and the management. It's a permissive climate and open-minded. A lot of laughter. There is no tension. It's stimulating to be a supervisor for these groups. They work during the supervision, always have issues that they want to raise, they share experiences with each other and are not judgemental, they can deal with challenges from each other and the supervisor. They don't have issues with their executives and trust their managers.

Group cards

There are different kinds of group cards to be used for various reasons. The group cards with several specific qualities (Better team spirit by Team card: This is me … and you?) may be used to help the group members get to know each other more closely (Bobacken & Pålsson, 2012). These cards are used after the supervisor has met the group a few times or whenever the group wants to have a little more focus on themselves. The cards aim at emphasising positive qualities in yourself and others. It usually requires a whole supervision session. Often the mood is inspiring. It's much appreciated to get so many positive comments by your colleagues. Some groups even take photographs of the cards to remember how much their colleagues appreciated one another.

Other group cards in the series can be more challenging when you should say something more fundamental about the group or how you feel in the group, your own approach, and experiences (This is what I think … and you?).

"If it was my client, I would …"

"If it was my client, I would …" is a method I use inspired by the experience from 18 years of participation in a dream group, where we analyse dreams using the method of Montague Ullman to understand the language of dreams. Ullman (1996) developed a group model to work with dreams. The model has a framework in which any dream can be heard. The dreamer maintains control the whole time by revealing only as much as she wants of sensitive issues or her private sphere. The task of the group is to offer support without pushing the dreamer, to respect the integrity of the dreamer and help her to understand her dream.

Together with the dreamer the group members actively explore the message of the dream by extracting meanings and feelings from within the dream images and making them their own. The leader of the group, based on her familiarity with the process, should secure the well-being of the dreamer, guide the group through the process and participate in the group as the other group members.

The dreamer is helped when the group is stimulated to discover aspects of the dream not easily noticed on her own. Group members need to train their ability to interpret to be able to give that help.

Using Ullman's dream method in supervision

Inspired by this method and my experience I have revised and adapted the method for supervision, to broaden the perspective on a supervisee's issue. She gains ideas and hear the thoughts and reflections of the group members on what she presented as a supervision question.

At the time of the interview I introduced the method that may permit the supervisee to find a range of perspectives, see her question from different angles and learn how others are thinking and what they might have done if they had been in a similar situation. With the method "if it was my client, I would ..." the supervisee doesn't need to hear thoughts and advice on what she should have done or must do that she perhaps already tried without any result.

The different steps in the supervision is like stages in a dream group.

The role and responsibility of the supervisor

The supervisor's role in this method is not much different from in any of the other methods. The supervisor is responsible for the structure and for keeping the limits. The task is to lead the group through the process, to be clear about the various steps that the group will follow and make sure that the group members stick to the agreed principles. The supervisor is part of the group and contributes thoughts and reflections based on the supervision question on the same terms as other members.

Stages in my method of supervision – summary

Stage I Who has a supervision question?

When the group has decided who will raise an issue the supervisee assisted by the supervisor will define the supervision question. The supervisor's task is to help the supervisee to formulate the supervision question. Most often it is dialogue between the supervisor and the supervisee. The supervisor maintains the structure and sets the limits to avoid the process developing into a general discussion of the problem. For more information on how the supervision question may be formulated, see part 4 in the book.

When the question has been defined according to the supervisee's needs, the supervisor writes the question on the board. The supervisee is asked how she wants to use the group.

Stage II Dialogue supervisee – supervisor – group

The supervisor and group members ask in-depth and clarifying questions or simply curious queries about how the supervisee finds herself with her client to understand as much as possible of the situation. The aim is to gain more details and a narrative based on the supervision question from the supervisee. The supervisor makes notes on the board on what the supervisee is sharing. It may be on the background of the client, the supervisee's task and responsibility in the matter, the client's current situation and need of assistance etc. The group members and supervisor also try to get an idea of how the supervisee is thinking and feeling, and what she has already done and want to do. What are the available resources and what might be the obstacles? On the board this is briefly noted in different colours.

I usually choose *black* for descriptions of the client's situation and background and any current difficulties in the matter (what is the client's problem, what sort of problem does the supervisee have to deal with in the current situation?).

In *red* I note down the supervisee's feelings and thoughts, responses to the client's situation and/or behaviour in the interview room.

In *blue* I make a note of what the supervisee says about her case and what she has already done in the current situation.

In *green* I write "solution", but there is no discussion of a solution at this stage, that comes in the final stage.

Stage III Regrouping

When the group members and supervisor have enough information on the current situation, the supervisor asks the supervisee to move out of the circle and face her chair away from the group. The others form a new circle. This makes it more difficult for them to turn to the supervisee and address her. From her new position the supervisee may undisturbedly listen to the group's conversation. The position also implies no one can observe the supervisee's body language or address thoughts and feelings to the supervisee, nor speak to her directly. Likewise, the supervisee is unable to observe anyone's body language.

Stage IV If it was my client, I would ...

In this stage each group member considers everything he has heard of the situation, sentiments, thoughts, and the issue itself and uses a first-person narrative to share what he would have done if it were his client.

The one starting says: If this was my client, I would ...

In this stage the supervisor keeps the structure and the process enabling everyone to talk from their own point of view, rather than telling what the supervisee ought to do. When a group member starts to talk about what he would do he is also getting supervision. If someone in the group finds it hard to assume the role of the supervisee, and instead would like to speak directly to her, it is the supervisor's task to help the group member to talk about what he would have done, felt, or thought if he was in the position of the supervisee, with the same issue and problem to solve. It requires an ability to sense the other person and for the moment step into her shoes, and on this basis enter a dialogue with the supervisor about your own sentiments, thoughts, and ideas about the direction to take, and how to proceed.

Every group member who has ideas on how he would act has the same dialogue with the supervisor. Finally, when everyone has shared their thoughts, the supervisor also asks: "if this was my client, I would ...". The supervisor shares her thoughts and feelings raised by the narrative: what she would do in the situation, how and with whom, but also why.

The short caption on the board helps everyone to remember the question, what kind of situation they are dealing with, what the supervisee feels and thinks and what they are trying to do to solve the problem at hand. The supervisor also makes brief notes on what each group member has said he would do and records her own thoughts.

Stage V Regrouping again

When everyone has said their piece, the supervisee is invited back into the circle. The supervisor asks the following questions: "While you were listening to us, what thoughts and feelings struck you? Is there anything that appeals to you from what you've heard? Did any new thoughts or ideas come up, any solutions? You know yourself, your own client, and your relationship best. From what you've heard you know what might be possible. Is it a combination of all this? Let's just hear what you want to say.

The supervisee shares his thoughts. The supervisor and group members can then ask in-depth and clarifying questions to get a better idea of and be able to understand what the supervisee has said. To be curious, to show respect and to accept without questioning or judging what the supervisee chooses to share are essential aspects at this stage.

Stage VI Summing up – Where to go from here?

The question and solutions of the group members and the supervisor are now up on the board. *The supervisor summarizes and asks the supervisee how he wish to proceed from here.* This is a process in which solutions are critically discussed and weighed together. The supervisee perhaps chooses an approach he will continue to process in upcoming sessions based on his current supervision question.

The supervision question might not anymore be relevant as originally framed. New thoughts and perspectives have surfaced, and the supervisee chooses to reframe and redefine his question.

There is room for discussing the advantages and consequences for the client and treatment that different alternatives entail. Which approach the supervisee chooses to embark on depends on several factors: the needs of the client, the theoretical framework of the supervisee, his room for action and his possibilities to apply the selected solution based on the client's resources and his own capacity.

Reflecting on the client's background, abilities and resources grants the supervisee some guidelines for his attitude to the client. The supervisee chooses his strategy considering the client's background and resources, and what the client wants help to resolve. It's not wrong to contrast the supervisee's idea of what the client needs against what he as a professional may offer. Supervision is a tool also to discover potential discrepancies between client's appreciation of her needs and the supervisee's assessment, and thus to find the optimal solution for the client.

The supervisee's theoretical knowledge and emotional commitment are important aspects when deciding on how to proceed. Theoretical knowledge helps in the analysis and understanding of the problem and relationship.

When the supervisee has decided on the alternative most suitable in the current situation, methods and techniques for implementation are discussed. Here the group and the supervisor may contribute with suggestions and their own experiences. When a supervisee becomes interested in a method he previously did not know, the supervisor may choose to introduce the method and its underlying theory and suggest ways the supervisee could apply it in the current situation. The supervisee is free to adopt what he believes is possible to realise and complete in his current work.

Stage VII What is your take home message?

In the last stage everyone expresses what they will take home from the session. At the next supervision meeting the supervisee can tell what results were achieved.

Writing on the board

A supervisor taking notes on a board or on a sheet of paper is of value both for the supervisee with a supervision question, and for the rest of the group. Some voices from supervision groups:

"The board gives an overview – we can see the question, how we are to answer it and that there are a variety of alternatives. The board helps to reduce the pressure. You see the goal. There is a clear path to tread."

"I like when you write on the board. Different colours make it clear what is what."

"You see your question and issues on the board and many different aspects to the question. That the work is complex become even more obvious. It becomes visual. Can see what's important. Someone conveys something that is useful to me. I find my calm in the supervision. Chance for reflection. It helps me develop my professional role."

"The board you use is fine. What we say becomes visible. It becomes clear. Things are put in order – when You write there is a break. Important to get the whole picture."

Model for working with unconscious processes

As a supervisee you have an opportunity to express a feeling you want to understand in process supervision. The supervisee wants to get "rid of" certain feelings and tries to find a professional attitude to avoid insulting or hurting a client. The supervisor and the supervision group are not to judge these feelings by their comments and interpretations.

To work with unconscious processes in the supervision an agreement is needed between the supervisor and the supervisee, a sort of contract, an established mandate. In dialogue with the supervisee the supervisor should now and again check if it's okay that they continue mutually exploring the feelings and corresponding unconscious emotions in focus.

The model is not based on the supervisor's interpretation of the emotion. Rather, in a 'dialogical dialogue', through questions and answers, the supervisor and supervisee try to find a common understanding of the emotion arising in meeting the client.

This model consists of different stages and the conversation is mostly between the supervisee and the supervisor. The supervisee do not have to answer questions by group members when something sensitive is discussed.

The dialogue as given in steps 1 to 8 below, begins with the supervisee describing his mood and finishes with a theoretical reflection, when the supervisor again describes the significant concepts, to let the supervisee himself link his mood to any of them.

Model using questions and answers

1. Can you describe your feeling? Try to put it into words

The supervisee tries to describe his feeling as detailed as possible. Sometimes several feelings come to life. The supervisor asks questions aiming at letting the supervisee choose the feeling that seems most important and on which he wants to focus. To put words on the feeling can sometimes be difficult and takes time. When the feeling which the supervisee wants to have in focus is defined the dialogue continues.

2. Where in your body do you locate the feeling?

The supervisee describes and specifies: Where in the body is this feeling? How does it feel? What is the intensity of the feeling?

3. In what situations might the feeling arise in relation to the client?

The questions are aimed at further investigating the settings when this feeling arises and to find out whether the supervisee at that point is aware of it. In what situations when meeting the client does this feeling arise? Are you aware of it when you speak to the client? Does the feeling show in a particular circumstance? Does it depend on the behaviour of the client? Does the feeling show when the client is talking about something specific?

4. Does the feeling occur in contact with any other client? If so, what do the clients have in common

After the supervisee has answered questions about the current client, the supervisor continues asking whether the same feeling may arise in meetings with other clients and, if so, is it of the same intensity. The supervisor's task is to help the supervisee to remember, to tell and compare.

"Do you sometimes feel the same with other clients?", "Does the feeling have the same quality and intensity together with other clients you are thinking of?", "What do these clients have in common?"

5. May the same feeling occur in your private life?

When the situation in the professional life of the supervisee has been elucidated you try together to identify whether the same feeling ever shows in his private life. Here, the supervisor needs only a short answer: yes or no. Even if the supervisee wants to reveal more it is the role and responsibility of the supervisor to assist in setting limits for what is said. If the answer is yes, the supervisor continues and asks of the feeling's quality and intensity. "Are these the same as towards the client?" The feeling might not have the same intensity here as it was described at the beginning of the dialogue, hence the supervisee changes his "yes" to a "no". It's not the same in his private life as with the client, even if it might have felt like that at first. The supervisor doesn't force any answers but asks the supervisee to remain with the feeling and explore it.

6. When the supervisee recognises the feeling in his private life

The supervisor continues with the process and the questions if the supervisee recognises the feeling also in his private life. The supervisor again emphasises, my questions should only be answered by yes or no. "Do you know towards whom in your private life these feelings might arise? And in what situations might the feelings show? You only need to answer yes or no." Usually the answer is that one knows i.e. yes. For the supervisor it's not important to know any more. If the supervisee wants to say more about what situation or person in his private life the supervisor should help him to say no more than is necessary for himself to be able to understand.

When the process has reached a point when the supervisee recognises the same feeling in his private life, and knows in what situation and with whom the feeling might show, the supervisor asks the question: "What do these individuals have in common, the client and the one in your private life?" Here a common feature or type of behaviour might be mentioned. Not a lot of information is required. The supervisor continues: "How did you solve this situation in your private life?" The most common answer is "not at all", or that he has "separated", "doesn't see the individual anymore", "continues to argue", "continues to be scared", "avoids contact with the individual" etc.

If the problem isn't resolved, if it's unconscious or conflicted it can easily be activated in the meeting with clients, when the situation with the client and the feelings that arise are reminiscent or have similarities to what has expired in private life. The supervisee can think about this and try to find solutions both for himself and for the relationship with the client.

Here the supervision ends, and the group is not invited to reflect on what has been revealed. Neither there are any comments. The supervisor continues explaining the meaning of the various unconscious concepts on which it may be relevant to reflect; see point 8 on theorisation.

When the supervisee does not recognise the feeling in his private life what he feels might be an expression of projective identification, which means that one carries the emotion of the client. If this is the case the supervisor changes focus and instead asks how that might affect the client.

7. Does the client feel the emotion and how does she express it?

The supervisor returns to the relationship with the client and together the supervisor and supervisee investigate how the client is affected. The supervisor asks the supervisee: "Do you think that the client can feel that emotion? How does the client express it? Could it be projective identification?" If the supervisee thinks the client can feel the emotion in focus but the client does not express it, then the supervisor again explains the concept and how projective identification may show in the relationship with the client. If the supervisee thinks that it's a matter of projective identification, then supervisor and supervisee together discuss ways in which the supervisee can return what is projected to the supervisee from the client. Belin (1993) calls this process to humanise the projected.

The supervisee can then ask the client how she feels in the situation she relates; conveying to the client: "Describe how you feel. I can listen. I'm here, I can stand hearing what you want to say. I'm with you." Even if it is not said directly the attitude is communicated in body language, the way of asking, and the tone in which the question is asked.

8. Theorizing: the supervisor defines relevant concepts of the unconscious process. Could you recognize your feeling in any of the described processes?

When the supervisee answers he recognise the feeling arising in his relation to his client from his private life, the supervisor gives a short description of what is meant by resonance, counter-transference and projective identification and asks the supervisee: "What do you think your feeling is an expression of? Could you relate the feeling to any of these concepts?" The supervisor is only interested in knowing if what was recognised can be a matter of projective identification to discuss how to return it to the client in a processed form without acting out. If it's a question of countertransference or resonance the supervisee doesn't have to say any more; Due to countertransference the supervisee has lost a sensible interest in his client who he sees as someone from his private life. In countertransference and resonance, the feeling does not disappear, but when the supervisee becomes aware of the origin of the feeling, he tries to adopt an attitude to the client which is positive for their relationship.

If the feeling is an expression of projective identification, it's common that the feeling of the supervisee is dissolved. There is even a sense of relief in the room and the feeling towards the client is altered. He can then feel more empathy and understanding for the client. Also if it is an issue of countertransference or resonance, there is a sense of relief. The supervisee understands that you cannot burden the client and your mutual relationship with your own personal history.

It may be that the feeling is an expression of both projective identification and countertransference and/or resonance.

Be aware that in certain situations a certain feeling may be a reasonable response to the client's behaviour. All feelings in the meeting with the client are not unconscious and everything does not need psychologising. You may be angry, upset, disappointed, frustrated, powerless and so on, in relation to your client/patient without that having anything to do with your past. If these feelings have been expressions of the unconscious and/or unprocessed experiences the processes in the supervision can lead to new experiences and an increased professionalism. It is then possible for the supervisee to use ongoing unconscious processes in a constructive way – the therapeutic relationship becomes healing for the client. The supervisor's task is to help the supervisee to the point where he begins to see that his personal experiences affect the process, and his own attitude can make a difference.

Reflection

Could you train your ability to recognise and know what a feeling express?
Yes, I think so. The professionals can themselves train their ability to observe and reflect on their feelings using the described stages. You may ask yourself the same questions. The greater your self-knowledge, the easier it becomes to recognise these feelings and how they are woven into your own history and experience.

Could all supervisors use this model? As a supervisor you cannot mechanically learn how to ask "the right questions" to arrive at what unconscious processes you are dealing with.

The supervisor's attitude and possibilities of creating work alliances and trust is a prerequisite for the supervisee to be able to discover his unconscious processes.

Other important circumstances are what is being played out in the interaction between the supervisee and the supervisor, the supervisee's capacity for reflection and level of self-knowledge as well as the supervisee's courage in deepening the relationship with the supervisor and having confidence in the supervisor and the group.

Model for working with parallel processes

A feeling arising within the supervisor could be investigated in the supervision to see whether it is an expression of a parallel process in the treatment and in the supervision. The model described in this section has been effective for me and the groups in which it has been applied. Together we have a common understanding of the emerging process. An approach focusing on exploring feelings and thoughts can be explained by using phenomenology, which recommends an exploration of experiences with focus on specific parts of the experience and certain feelings without any theoretical speculation.

This model has six different stages.

Stage 1: The supervisor's inner experience

In this stage the supervisor identifies an emotion or a blocking. For example, when the supervisor experiences difficulties in relation to the supervisee or when she can't find a way to continue the supervision process. The supervisor records the triggered emotion and thoughts in her notebook.

If the mood continues for more than 10–15 minutes the supervisor asks the group to discuss the presented case to get as much clarity as possible. The supervisor encourages further discussion by asking: "Do you have any questions? Is there anything else you want to know about this matter?" By engaging the group in the process, the supervisor has an opportunity for a moment to distance herself and reflect on her experience and feelings. The "inner supervisor" and questions asked by the group members may create new perspectives for the supervisor and offer a chance to put new questions or find a new way to continue working with the supervision process.

Stage 2: To "freeze" the situation – here and now

When it did not help to engage the supervision group the supervisor "freezes" the situation to overcome her own feelings and difficulties, or her own blocking. The supervisor freezes the situation by saying for example:

"We can stop here for a moment. Let's freeze this situation between me and the supervisee. Let's adopt a meta-position. Describe, without analysing, interpreting, or guessing, how you are experiencing the dialogue. Share with me what you feel, your experience of the dialogue and the feelings and thoughts that came to you while you were listening. What would you say happened?"

In accordance with the phenomenological idea of placing one's earlier knowledge "in parenthesis" during the supervision, the supervisor can emphasise the importance of every group member isolating his own feelings and thoughts as a pure phenomenon and clearly express his experience of the situation. This phase, in which the situation is frozen, is the beginning of an externalisation process, that is to name one's feelings and thoughts. When we express ourselves in words, listen to ourselves and others and write on the board, we simultaneously use more than one sense. We don't only hear what others say, what we say also becomes visible to everyone.

Stage 3: Visualise everyone's experience of the process

In this stage of externalisation every group member, including the supervisor, talks about their feelings and thoughts without interpreting or explaining them. The supervisor writes what every participant says on the board, making it visible to everyone. It's important that everyone describes his feelings and thoughts without being influenced by the supervisor or any guidelines. When all have described their feelings and thoughts it's the turn of the supervisor to describe hers. The supervisor's role in this phase is through dialogue to help every group member identifying his feelings and thoughts.

According to Husserl in Kordeš (2008) placing our theoretical knowledge and convictions within parenthesis means:

The rule: don't explain; describe! This is the most important methodological guideline in phenomenological research. This call may seem simple at first glance, but its application is complex and requires a well-developed capacity to reflect and the ability to only describe observations and experiences without placing them in any kind of theoretical framework or clarifying them. (Transl. p.51)

Phenomenological dialogue entails that the investigator does not lead the dialogue in a desired direction, but rather maintain a position of "not-knowing". The more we free ourselves of our ideas and attitudes, the more space we create for new knowledge. Questions are supports by which we show our presence and interest. The phenomenological dialogue is a technique of self-exploration, the true explorer is the one who answers. The individual asking questions is only a support in this exploration of this inner perceptual room (Kordeš, 2008).

Stage 4: Back to the supervisee

In this stage the supervisor asks the supervisee who has presented the supervision question to observe all notes recorded on the board. Focus now returns to the supervisee. "Look at all the comments on the board and tell us which ones you consider to best describe your *client's feelings, thoughts and reflections.*" The supervisor circles in a colour the comments the supervisee identifies as typical for his client, and then asks for example: "Now look at what's written again. What of that written on the board might *characterise you and your work with your client*? What do you think or feel yourself in working with the client? You can also choose the already encircled alternatives." When the supervisee identifies the comments corresponding to his feelings the supervisor circles these in a new colour, and if something is already circled a second circle is added. The supervisor continues with the question: "Which of these comments, including those already encircled, might be said to *describe your relationship with the client?*" These are marked in a third colour and if any of the comments are already circled, a new circle in the third colour joins the ones already there. Finally, some comments are circled in one colour, others in two and some in three colours, while some are not circled at all.

During this phase it may become clear which of the feelings, processes, moods, or difficulties in the supervision situation are expressions of a parallel process – i.e. which ones correspond to what is happening in the treatment and which ones may be expressions of other processes, either in the treatment or in the supervision. Certain feelings and thoughts that have occurred in the supervision process may remain unmarked. These not encircled comments may, however, generate ideas on how the relationship and work with the client could be developed.

Stage 5: Theorizing and inter-subjectivity

In this stage everyone in the group observes what has been written on the board and what has been encircled. Everyone reflects on what has been written and creates with the assistance of the supervisor a theoretical framework for the supervision process and the identified parallel process. This is an important stage of the supervision. It's part of learning about and gaining an understanding of the treatment process and the supervision process, also about the role you play in these processes. The concept of inter-subjectivity, which means that something grows out of groupwork, and cooperation based on encounters and experiences, as well as taking shape in the form of parallel processes, can help the supervisor and supervision group on a meta-level to gain an understanding and an overview of the situation.

Stage 6: How could the work with the client continue

In this stage the supervisee formulates ideas and thoughts on what might be the next stage of the treatment and how it can be achieved. The other participants in the group also express their thoughts on how they would have continued the work if it was their client. The supervisor only contributes ideas if no one in the group has expressed a similar thought. When everyone has put forward their ideas and discussed pros and cons, the supervisor turns to the supervisee who presented the issue: "Now you have heard our thoughts on what we would have done if it was our client. Only you know yourself and your client. Now that you've listened to our thoughts: what idea, combination of ideas, or new idea that you've had would be most suitable to use in your continued work with the client? You only need to choose the ideas which seem most useful to you and your client in the current situation and which it would be possible to apply."

To facilitate the supervisor might ask questions such as: "How do you intend to move forward? What will you focus on? Is this what you want to do? What potential problems do you foresee in taking the work forward?"

Žorga writes that according to Kolb:

… learning is a holistic process which comprises the integrated work of the whole organism – thoughts, feelings, beliefs and behaviour. This is precisely what happens in the supervision process when the supervisee adapts and integrates new-won knowledge with practical skills, perspectives and patterns of behaviour. (Žorga, 2009, s. 37)

When the supervisee returns to his workplace, he applies what he has learned and what might be effective in the given situation and for the client. The actual implementation is dependent on the supervisee's level of competence, the client's ability and motivation to receive the offered solution. The flexibility and resources of the organisation has a bearing on whether what has been discussed in the supervision is possible to accomplish.

Could all supervisors use this model?

Every stage in this supervision model has its own structure and prepares for the next stage. It's an interactive process at two levels: the process within the supervisor that can be observed at a meta-level, and the process the supervisor observes between herself and the supervisee in the supervision group. The interactive process is about how you know, how you choose and how you act.

The model can be applied in many different situations, but some supervisors may not feel quite comfortable with the concept of parallel processes if they don't use or accept psychodynamic thinking. Obstacles and blocks that might be explained by an unconscious parallel process may therefore remain undiscovered or unresolved both in treatment and in the supervision dialogue. The supervisee who, for example, works within cognitive behavioural therapy, solution-focused therapy or system therapy doesn't directly work with unconscious processes, or with parallel processes, in the way described here. This supervision model may be used differently depending on context and the approach the supervisor demands in the supervision process. More details on the model can be found in Cajvert, 2011 and Cajvert, 2013.

Silent positioning – Life Staging

In the supervision I sometimes introduce Life Staging, a method that the psychologist, certified psychotherapist, and supervisor Elisabeth Wollsén developed (www.lifestaging.se). The supervision groups in which I have used the method have been appreciative. They have often gained new perspectives on their work, their client, or the situation. Furthermore, Life Staging may help them to better understand their own family and themselves. To observe a silent positioning and 'hear' how individuals experience their position through their body language may also promote empathy for the supervisee in focus, the positioner. There's a difference explaining a case in words, talking about your own problems, situation, and feelings, and physically undertaking group work where the body is the instrument giving 'voice' and 'words' to thoughts and feelings when you are in a specific positioning. I am presenting the method as Wollsén herself describes it, along with the idea and theory underpinning it.

Life Staging is an alternative supervision format focusing creativity and personal development. The method utilizes the whole person, in all its uniqueness and rich colouring, by liberating what might otherwise be silenced by norms on how to behave or what you should do. The method challenges traditional supervision formats focusing largely on understanding, explaining, and solving verbally. The analysis of problems and how things should be resolved is not in focus in Life Staging; rather it exposes the values, wishes, fears and preconceptions of the complexity of life. The method encourages the supervisee to let go of psychological lingo and theoretical explanatory models, preconceived knowledge, and possibly biased simplifications.

Life Staging can be described as a type of representation in which all are involved in creating the content by alternately observing and engaging in interplay. Using the scene the supervisee creates, dilemmas and questions can be defined, be more visible and at the same time more complex. The original, first scene is a sort of outline which the participants then help to develop into a richer image by showing new scenes.

Ideas underpinning the supervision model Life Staging

Through Life Staging/ Positioning you gain access to a different kind of information, practice other tasks and develop further knowledge and skills compared to traditional supervision. Moving around in the room, adopting body positions and improvising together create a unique atmosphere in the supervision group, that the supervisees often bring back to their workplace. "Elements of humour always show in the positioning which positively affects the atmosphere during the supervision. Supervisees using the method describe a feeling of increased energy, improved cooperation and they become less polarised", writes Wollsén.

The positioning proceeds from a position of 'not-knowing' and non-verbal activities. All participants are active and help each other to create a variety of scenes, free of values and any pressure to perform. Nothing is right or wrong. According to Wollsén the main purpose of Life Staging is to challenge prejudice and develop relational skills, courage, and the ability to improvise – to practise trust and presence. The method brings out the original, personal and creative in each participant. The participants develop skills that you cannot "study" to learn and are not easily developed if you simply talk about the situation or what it generates. When verbal elements occur, it is in very plain language that facilitates participants to express themselves more personally and spontaneously. By taking part in Life Staging you become more observant, more aware of your notions about yourself and others. You need to be "empty" to see. An insight grows that you need others to see the "whole picture" and that interaction and cooperation is what decides how a meeting develops.

Silent positioning in practice

The supervision session starts as usual by someone in the group wanting to raise an issue and ready to be in focus. If the supervisee chooses silent positioning, he is not to say either what the question is, or whom or what is to be included in the question.

Thus, even the supervisor does not know which issue to be addressed.
- "You would like to do a silent positioning?"
- The supervisor here needs to clarify to the supervisee that he is not to describe his dilemma or what the positioning is about. Everyone in the room is then asked to stand up to create energy and movement. The supervisor focus on the positioner and stands beside him during the process, except during the first scene.
- The supervisor then asks the supervisee to consider who or what objects should be part of the scene and select the group members who should represent the various aspects, individuals or phenomena – reminding: don't to think too much!
- The supervisor also reminds him that a person should be selected to represent the positioner and, in this role, to be part of the scene.
- The positioner is asked to give instructions, non-verbal, using body language and gestures to direct each person: how they should stand or sit, the direction of their gaze, posture, facial expression, gestures and so on. Instructions are also given to the person who will represent the positioner in the scene.
- "You position the persons in relation to each other based on the idea that you have of what you want to explore more closely. You can use the whole room as a scene and everything in the room to assist you!"
- The positioner is then asked to observe the scene at some distance, if necessary, adjusting, strengthening and clarifying further.
- Once the positioner is satisfied with the set-up, the supervisor takes him to one side and stands with him to observe the image/scene together.
- The supervisor thereafter turns to the persons in the scene and asks them to stay in their positions for a few seconds and sense what it feels like to be part of the scene, to be in contact with themselves and their feelings.

- In the next step the supervisor gives instructions to the positioned members in the scene to do whatever they feel like based on their positions in the first scene, still using no words. For example, they can move freely across the scene, change their facial expressions, act in some way. This makes a new constellation possible and already gives an altered view, a new perspective on the relationship between the participants in the scene.
- The supervisor halts the process after a few minutes and asks the individuals in the scene to say something by giving the instruction "Voices". At this point each person should share, in plain language, what he has experienced, felt or thought since first being positioned until the present scene, altered by his and the others' movements. "What happened to you, why did you choose to do what you did, what did you feel in front of the others?" etc. No psychological explanations or psychological analysis should be attempted. Also, no guesses on who you are portraying in the positioning. If someone did attempt to do so the supervisor interrupts by repeating the questions.
- When everyone in the scene has shared their experiences, the supervisor asks the positioner if he wants to question any other person in the scene, to get a more complete picture.
- It's then possible to continue building the scene in various ways.
- The supervisor asks the positioner: "Would you like to try a new scene, or would you like someone on the stage to perform the next scene? Again, using no words." Sometimes the positioner wants to stage a new scene, or someone among the positioned is asked for suggestions on the next scene, or perhaps the positioner would like to try both alternatives. All these new scenarios give new constellations, voices and perspectives. Finally, the positioner is satisfied and does not want to try any more scenes.
- When the different scenes have been completed and the positioner says that he is satisfied with what he has seen and gained from the process, the supervisor asks if the positioner would like to reveal who or what the participants represent, still without revealing what it's all about. Based on this, further voices may be added by the positioned members about their 'character', their position and experience in the scene.
- Before everyone sits down in the circle it's important that the individuals who have taken part in the scene shake off the role that they have played. This is done together by helping each other to 'pull off' their role figures, (so called de-rolling).
- The supervisor now emphasises that the positioner is in focus and sits with him a little to one side and makes clear to the others that they are not to interrupt

the dialogue between the supervisor and positioner. The supervisor then asks the positioner: "What did you experience from the moment you began the positioning and through all the scenes? What did you see, what happened to you, how do you feel and think now about what has happened, what you have seen and heard?"

- The positioner is also asked if he wants to discuss what the positioning was about. The supervisor's task now is to make sure that the positioner stays with what has happened during the positioning process and not start to talk and give information based on their previous idea of his dilemma.
- A question is also asked whether the positioner wants to hear the reflections of others in the group. Sometimes the positioner is satisfied, he might already be involved in an emotional process and wants to avoid hearing additional perspectives on what he already has arrived at himself. In case reflections are offered by others, they are encouraged to describe ways in which they recognise themselves in their professional role dealing with the same dilemma. Here, they should not give advice to the positioner or analyse, they should rather refer to themselves and their own experiences.

A summary of how to perform life staging

Positioning
- The supervisee: I want to have space – I want to do a silent positioning
- The supervisor: Important to remember:
  - Show without words who should take part in the scene. Position these persons in relation to one another, based on the image you have
  - Don't forget to include someone as representative of yourself.
  - Remember; do not use words. Do not reveal the story behind the positioning.

Scene 1
- The supervisor to the positioner: Observe the scene at some distance. Adjust without using words. Refine and strengthen using facial expressions and gestures. The positioner thereafter leaves the scene and observes at some distance together with the supervisor.
- The supervisor to the persons in the scene: Remain in the image that has been created. Be still for 5–7 seconds and explore what you are feeling.

- Next you can do whatever takes your fancy, a movement, no words. A new scene is created, an altered image.
- The supervisor interrupts after a few minutes and asks each person in the positioning:
  What happened to you?
  - What did you experience?
  - Why did you choose to do as you did?
  - Describe in simple and everyday language. Try not to think too much!
- The supervisor asks the positioner: Are you satisfied? Would you like to try another scene? Would you like to ask someone else to try a new scene?
  In that case who would you like to make a new scene.

Scene 2
- The selected positioner sets up positions based on the information in scene 1.
- Without using words he shows who are to take part in the scene. Directs positions, facial expressions and gestures.
- The positioned are told to remain in their positions for 5–7 seconds and then do whatever they feel like doing, again without using words.
- The supervisor interrupts after a few minutes and each person is again asked to describe:
  - What did you experience?
  - Why did you choose to do as you did?
  - Describe in simple and everyday language. Try not to think too much!

Scene 3
- If the positioner wants to try out more scenes, the same procedure is repeated as above. When the positioner is satisfied the supervisor asks them:
  - Would you like to explain who the participants represent? Still without revealing the dilemma.
  - More comments may be offered by those positioned.
  - All are de-rolled and sit in a circle.
The supervisor sits down together with the positioner.
  - Take your time now.
  - Describe what you have experienced.
  - What did you see? Anything new?
  - Anything confirmed?
  - What does this do with you?

The positioner is then asked if he would like to hear more from the group.

The supervisor turns to the others in the group and asks about resonance and reflection:

What did you see? What affected you? Could it be connected to something that you recognise in yourself? What will you take away from here, did the scenes carry you anywhere?

The positioner thereafter, without anyone interfering, gives his own narrative based on what he has experienced and the session ends.

The supervisor – 'an artistic director'

Wollsén argues that the supervisor acts as an artistic director by activating dormant skills and abilities; the supervisees become more daring, more observant and can find their unique personal expression. The supervisor maintains the structure and steers the process making it comfortable for the positioner and participants, by giving clear instructions, brief changes of the scene and verbal directions, in all encouraging richer images and narratives supporting the supervisee in resolving his supervision question. More about Elisabet Wollsén's model can be found at www.lifestaging.se.

Taping with Playmobil® figures in supervision

Taping is a method developed by Martin Soltvedt (2005) in working with children in therapy. The materials are painted wooden figures that parents and children use to embody their life situation, their network, internal or external conflicts. Professionals in different fields use this method for exploratory work and treatment.

Having pursued various courses and attending meta-supervision by the certified psychotherapist and supervisor Christina Löwenborg I sometimes use taping with Playmobil® figures in my supervision. The Löwenborg (2013, 2016, 2017) supervision model is inspired by three theoretical orientations: *taping*, as developed by Martin Soltvedt (2005), *schema therapy*, developed by Jeffrey Young (Young & etc, 2003) and *psychodrama*, developed by Peter Felix Kellerman (1992). According to Löwenborg these directions are to a high degree compatible in a supervision context. All have a connection to play and spontaneity. What in taping is externalised by figures on a table as a scene, is embodied in psychodrama on a scene and in schema therapy by visualisation on an inner scene. Löwenborg argues that taping, psychodrama, and the schema therapy model integrate the function of the cognitive analysis with an immediate emotional experience coupled with active participation, i.e. an integration of head, heart and action. This working method makes dialogue visual and concrete; the supervisee can create a scenario using figures and symbols, which represent a situation. The narrative in this way becomes a visual creation.

Assisted by this integrative model the narrative simultaneously takes on a from-the-outside and a -within perspective. Thus, it allows an illustration of both an outer and inner reality. The image gives a bird's eye view on those involved and their relationship to one another, at the same time making visible ongoing affects activated within them. The method can be applied in many different situations offering a representation of a problem of some kind, a conflict, a vision, someone's story or two contradictory stories, the network around a person, an inner conflict, or a trauma.

Löwenborg emphasizes the advantage of using a concrete, visual and representative methodology in a supervision context making the supervisee's ideas visible, clarified and concrete. By using such a tangible working method, you create a shared idea – everyone present has the same image to which they can relate. In the supervision it is advantageous if the represented situation created on the table kindles the commitment of the group, enabling each one to connect to his own experience. A strong sense of participation improves cooperation between those involved and is a good basis for the continued process in the supervision.

In supervision complex issues may be tackled. As a situation can be built and shown from different aspects that may influence the outcome, you get an overview of the given scenario and an understanding of the process. The concrete narrative in the image gives a sense of reality and increases the emotional temperature.

The model is characterised by the mobile scene of figures on the table. The story may take place in the past, the present, or future. It may show parallel occurrences and it may simultaneously show an outer and an inner reality. The figures can be moved back and forth to portray an event. All this facilitate reflections and exploration of thoughts and ideas. In the supervision all participants can be invited and present their thoughts and ideas in a concrete way.

The model uses Playmobil® figures of various age, ethnicity and gender. The figures have moveable parts which can be useful in the supervision. By turning their heads, arms and legs the figures' expressions and attitudes can be accentuated and the relation between them become clearer. The relationships between the figures can be made more distinct by concrete actions: they can stand close to or far from one another, they can turn toward or away from each other, depending on what is being portrayed in the scene.

Löwenborg uses figures together with symbols which makes the story more comprehensible and meaningful. The symbols can help making the situation clearer and allowing emotions to be expressed. It could be a twisted tangle placed between persons to illustrate tricky and controversial relations. It might be a stone symbolising a weight, perhaps of grief or depression. A heart can symbolise trust or security in a relationship. A telephone can symbolise that there is communication and a fence the opposite. To express feelings and forces between those involved, wild and tame animals may be used. A bull can symbolise forcefulness and a little rabbit can symbolise fear. A tortoise can show how a person crawls into their shell to protect themselves and a snake can represent unpredictability. The narrator chooses symbols expressing the subjective idea to be staged on the scene. The story is supported and emotionally loaded by concrete symbols. The concrete narrative in images gives the experience a realistic sense and the assembled image stays in memory.

In the concluding phase connections are made between what takes place in the scene and what is occurring in real life. The focus moves from the emotionally lived experience to cognitive processes, how the experiences can be transposed to reality and how the generated knowledge can be generalised to include everyone present. Finally, the core aspects are integrated: head, heart and action. You can read more on Löwenborg's model at www.lowenborg.eu.

Evaluation as intervention

I often bring up the method "evaluation as intervention" in the supervision, for example, when a supervision question concerns a supervisee being stuck at work with a client and asking for advice or ideas on how to move on. Such instants have different names in the therapeutic literature such as for example plateau, deadlock or stagnation. There are also different interpretations on what may be the cause, for example resistance, or the client not being motivated.

Evaluation as intervention can be of assistance in the ongoing work, to get out of a deadlock and/or to find out if the treatment has any effect and is meaningful – without interpreting the situation. It may also help the therapist to be in touch with her own perceptions and how these direct the therapeutic relationship or directs ideas about the right decisions and measures to be taken. This model is a way to facilitate self-reflection for both the client and therapist and can function as a "supervision" in the continued contact and course.

When can evaluation as intervention be used?

Here are some common situations in which evaluation as intervention could be used:
- If a plateau has been reached in treatment
- If the client again and again fails to show up
- If the client indicates that the therapeutic conversation doesn't help or doesn't create the desired change
- If the client and therapist have different opinions on the potential of their dialogues to make a change
- If the therapist wants to emphasise the client's own resources and focus on his participation and his ability to change his circumstances in life
- To encourage the client to look more closely at the therapeutic work, express his opinion on the process of which he is a part
- To give the client a chance to take his own initiative in the continuing process and direction
- To gain a sharper idea of what the client wants, if he wants something the therapist has not been able to discover or paid attention to
- If the therapist does not know where she finds herself in the treatment process.

Quantification & dialogue based on past – today – future

Evaluation as intervention starts on a scale from 0 till 10. Such a scale is a very common tool in therapeutic work. First, the evaluation should be originating from an overarching question which has been a focus of the sessions. It must be measurable. An overarching question might be: "I want to have greater self-confidence", "I want to communicate in a different way with my wife", "I want to dare to say no", "We don't communicate with each other in our family" and so on.

Scaled questions are used for instance in solution-focused brief therapy. Korman and Söderquist (1994) write that scaled questions are useful in clarifying the wishes and desires of the client. The questions allow follow-up and carry the conversation forward. The client and therapist may also gain clarity on how the client experiences his situation and change.

To make it clear and comprehensible for the client the therapist uses a board or a notepad writing down the scale marked from 0 to 10. She explains: 0 is when it is at its worst and 10 when it works or feels at its best. 10 can also represent the declared goal of the treatment, how one wants to see one's situation or how one wants to feel after the therapy.

If the therapist is working with a family or a couple, they can make a scale for the whole family or the couple or make an individual scale for each person. It is up to the therapist and/or client what will be observed and attended to, or which processes the therapist wants to focus. First a little about the scale and dialogue to be pursued with the client.

On the scale from one to ten you may enter figures for THEN, TODAY and FUTURE (see Figure 5.1).

Figure 5.1 Scale as a tool in evaluation
THEN – at the first contact before we began working with your issue, where were you on a scale 0 to 10? Tentative answer 2, shown in the diagram

0	1	2	3	4	5	6	7	8	9	10
		THEN								

THEN refers to how the situation was before the client began the treatment, for example at the first meeting. The client gives a figure from 0 till 10 to represent what he felt in the beginning. The client should plainly describe how he felt and thought and what he was doing at that time. The therapist begins a dialogue on feelings, thoughts, behaviour, and events. The purpose is to be concrete and detailed about something that has occurred or has been felt. You should be able to compare to how things are now, today. By concretising it becomes easier to note any improvements, deterioration, or if the situation is unchanged. The therapist compares how the client now describes the situation and how he described the same situation at the start of the treatment. It's an advantage if the therapist has a good memory, or at least has read her notes before the evaluation, to have a dialogue with the client in case he describes the situation in a different way or don't remember. The therapist can remind the client of the earlier description but not persuade the client or force him to remember the same as the therapist. The client should only confirm the therapist's version of events if it accords with his own.

Figure 5.2 Scale as a tool in evaluation

TODAY – where are you today on a scale 0 to 10? Tentative answer 4, shown in the diagram below.

0 1	2 3	4 5 6	7	8 9 10
		TODAY		

TODAY refers to the client's description of how he finds himself today. First, he gives a figure which the therapist notes on the scale and then he describes as detailed as possible his feelings and thoughts today. How does the client do this?

There are three alternatives the client may speak of: it's better today, a higher figure than THEN, it's unchanged, or a lower figure than THEN. Regardless of what the client replies the therapist asks the same questions on improvement, no change or worsening. It's important that the therapist does not steer the process, but rather seeks to find out what the client feels and how he describes how the treatment has affected his present condition today.

The therapist continues and asks *what* is better, worse, or different. When this has been tackled in a concrete way the therapist asks what and who has contributed to this condition:

- How did he (i.e. the client) contribute
- how did the environment and/or family contribute
- how did the therapist or their meetings contribute?

The therapist asks these same questions regardless of how the client has answered on alternatives 1, 2 or 3 (see the scale). Especially if there is a feeling of a worsening or an unchanged situation it's important to discuss what is worse, how the client himself has contributed to it, what impact the environment has had and what the therapist has contributed. The therapist gains insight into her own contribution, which may has made it worse for the client. It's important that the therapist does not get offended or upset if the client says he is feeling worse. By follow-up questions the therapist may find out if there is something he might have contributed, or whether a worsening described by the client is a natural phase in the therapeutic process. It's not unusual that the client after a period of treatment observes feeling worse as the emotions he tries to express are activated or recharged. Especially if the client uses alternatives 2 or 3 the therapist should be using follow-up questions to assist the client in elaborating and comparing THEN and TODAY. Helped by the therapist it's not unusual for the client to see that things have changed although his initial response was no change. In that case, together, you might more closely explore what makes the everyday experience or reality seem unchanged. Such a dialogue may create insights that the client shares, and that are not left open to interpretation.

The client experiencing matters to be worse may for example be a result of certain secrets or lies being exposed during the treatment. The therapist may unconsciously have taken sides with some family member or expressed an opinion which has reinforced the conflict, leading to a deterioration. The conversation may also have touched issues that was not the purpose of the treatment, and which the client hadn't dared to mention. In this way the therapist could correct specific mistakes and become aware of being biased or of counter-transference mechanisms that may unintentionally upset the client.

The evaluation offers an opportunity to change the direction of the dialogue and correct misconceptions and mistakes. In the same way the therapist can help the client to become aware of a change which he has overlooked – the feeling may be the same, but the situation may be entirely different. The change that has been overlooked can create a sense of hope and in such a case the evaluation has had a therapeutic effect.

Figure 5.3 Scale as a tool in evaluation
FUTURE – where would you like to be on a scale 0 to 10 six months from now?
Tentative answer 6, shown in the diagram below

0 1	2 3	4 5 6	7	8 9 10
FUTURE				

The FUTURE refers to how you should continue. The therapist can deal with this in two ways. She can ask the client how far along the scale he wants to reach, or herself offer a suggestion and indicate that on the scale. If the client has seen an improvement from 2 to 4 it's good pedagogic practice and encouraging if the therapist does not indicate any figure above 6 in case she suggests a figure representing the future for the client (Figures 5.1 – 5.3).

Personally, I never use the 10. It's in some way the maximum and optimal state which I would rather let the client reach toward in his life ahead. If the client says that he finds himself at 9, I will use 9 ½ to carry on a dialogue about the future.

The future dialogue would then refer to how matters may appear in a concrete sense and what the client needs to get to 9 ½. How would that feel? How would the client then think about his problem? What does the client want to do? The discussion may cover:

• what he can and wants to continue of what worked
• what helped and how can he use his experience
• what will be required of himself and how may he contribute
• what is required from his peers and family
• what are his expectations of the therapist, what can the therapist do and contribute?

In the last point the therapist may gain information on whether the client's wishes are realistic: whether she can, wants and is allowed to satisfy the client's wishes She might also discover that the client does not know what the therapy can achieve: for example that she can offer more than what the client may be aware of. The therapist realises the client's expectations and can compare with her own expectations or possibilities. The client may also want to continue the process on his own and in such a case the evaluation has been useful for ending the therapy. The client may find that he can cope without the therapist, and perhaps the relationship is ended earlier than planned. The therapeutic effect is to promote hope in the client, to increase self-confidence and improve his self-image. The client attains an image of himself as not being as bad as he had thought because the treatment was successful more quickly than anticipated.

Evaluation as intervention helps the client to discover his own resources and abilities and gain an insight that he himself contributed to the change. If the client discovers his own resources, he will be a motivated and may get a desire, almost a longing, to try out his own strengths, his wings, on his own initiative. It's enticing to be self-reliant and function in everyday life in a satisfactory way without help from a therapist, albeit supported by experiences gained from therapy sessions.

Reflection

Evaluation as intervention can be used by the therapist when dealing with clients who have lost hope of attaining change. When he has lost all hope of real change, help is needed to help him realise that he still may be changed. By detailing what has been and how it is today, and by the therapist writing this on the board, the client realises that he has changed although he does not feel that. Change is possible and awakens hope. The written activates more senses than when you only talk. It's useful for clients who are more visual than aural.

Many therapists have used evaluation as intervention in a variety of therapies and it has generally been the same positive experience as it has been for the clients. Therapists state that it's good to have something tangible to focus, especially if a session has been chaotic. The method makes it easier to maintain a common thread and there is a structure to follow. As a therapist you also get confirmation of having done something well – or not.

Some therapists had noted that their client felt worse, but through this intervention found that they had misunderstood the situation and to the contrary it appeared that their client was satisfied. The therapist thus gained insight; his opinion was not in line with that of the client, which may have taken the therapeutic process in an unfavourable direction for the client.

In this model the client is active and participates more. It also becomes clearer what the client wants of the therapist. The method demonstrates the importance of discussing content. It requires skill on the therapist's part to have a dialogue and ask questions on the level of both content and process. Active listening and use of "the Socratic dialogue" make it possible for the client to reflect and gain insights, and the same is true for the therapist.

This model can also be used in supervision to evaluate development.

6. Feedback & Evaluation in supervision

FEEDBACK and EVALUATION are important components of supervision. Both activities offer an opportunity to change the direction of the mutual work and thereby avoid long, drawn-out, and unproductive processes. Both help you to discover and identify experiences and conceptions not consistent with actual events in the supervision – allowing misconceptions to be tracked and tackled, thereby avoiding unresolved conflicts to be transferred to a new supervisor, or another supervision group.

Disagreements in a group or dissatisfaction or disappointment with a superior are sometimes projected on a supervisor. An assessment may facilitate detection of an area of dissatisfaction and clarify its causes.

Feedback

Feedback includes responses or reactions to what a supervisee or supervisor has said or done during a supervision session. Feedback may be given to increase awareness of what you are doing, saying, or how you behave in the professional context, how you are perceived and experienced by others and/or the effect on others of what you say or do. This kind of awareness is important in a profession where you are dealing with other people. How is feedback to be given without threatening the self-esteem of anyone?

Feedback should be given with respect and in the form of a dialogue, especially if something needs to be improved, developed and/or changed in the work, behaviour, attitude, or way of communicating. Constructive feedback (Eide & Eide, 2012) is characterized by how it supports the person in what he has achieved and should focus what needs to be improved.

Feedback should be clear and concrete. How feedback is received also depends on how it is communicated. Feedback is given through open-ended questions and should always begin with what is working well, what the individual has managed to do, before bringing up aspects to be developed or changed. It should always be delivered as a personal 'I message' (Gunnarsson, 2014). Gunnarsson describes feedback as:

a) appreciative and supportive of what is being done well
b) remedial, constructive suggestions on what might be done better

Feedback is intended to contribute to the development of an another. To avoid negative consequences of feedback the relationship must be based on trust. It's "about helping others to understand that they are visible, interesting and meaningful" (a.a., p. 14). Gunnarsson writes about some areas which are particularly suitable for feedback and that I believe are relevant to the supervisor in relation to the supervisee. These different areas correspond to and are like a supervision question or issues group members together reflect on during supervision.

- *Interplay/cooperation*: How does the interaction function regarding the target group, colleagues, co-workers, and the supervisor? What works less well and how should it be developed?
- How does the supervisee *perform at work and in his work tasks*?
- How does the supervisee *behave*: What is his attitude to the group in focus, towards colleagues, co-workers, and the supervisor: What does he do that is appreciated, and how? In what way does his behaviour need to change and regarding which target group? How can he be helped by the supervisor in changing his behaviour?
- Is this type of behaviour *in line with the values of the organisation*: What he does in relation to the target group – is that in line with how you should behave in that workplace?
- Does the supervisee himself ask for any feedback – What? May the supervisor provide what he requests? Is the supervisee ready to receive it? How does he use the advice?

It's not unusual for colleagues to give each other feedback during the supervision. In my experience most colleagues and work groups are respectful to one another when they give feedback and have a tone and approach that makes it easier for the person in focus to receive the feedback. The supervisor can give feedback on her own initiative or when the group member or the group asks for it. When feedback is given the supervisor discusses the issue at hand and not the individual.

Feedback from the supervisor is the supervisor's response to and understanding of what the supervisee is doing. By listening to and backing the supervisee, the supervisor offers him support and makes him feel less vulnerable. Respect and clarity by the supervisor are attitudes that enables the individual in focus not becoming defensive or even rejecting feedback. The supervisor's feedback is aimed at helping the supervisee to reflect on what he is doing and should not be communicated or seen as criticism. It should make the supervisee willing to change what needs to be changed. The supervisor judges when and how to react by feedback.

Evaluation

Evaluation may be done at different occasions and for different purposes. The first evaluation is performed when everyone in the group has had supervision on one case, or at the latest at the end of the first term. For groups with only a limited number of sessions per term at least seven or eight meetings are required before it's time to evaluate how well the supervision has functioned.

The purpose of the first evaluation is to allow each participant to share his opinion on how the supervision has been and whether it has achieved set goals and met expectations. The group and the supervisor have a new opportunity to consider whether they want to continue the supervision. New evaluations can then be done at the end of each term. The appropriate head of the organisation is invited once a year to take part in the evaluation.

Sometimes the supervisor may evaluate after each supervision session. The purpose is to review and reflect on the process together, especially for groups having supervision only once a month or on a few occasions during the term.

If there are problems in the supervision the supervisor can ask questions such as: "What did you expect? How did it work? How should we continue? What needs to be changed?"

Personally, I almost always use the last supervision session of the term for an assessment, and especially if a long break will follow. Sometimes the supervisees or the supervisor leaves the final supervision worried or being dissatisfied. In such a case this may only be raised at the first session after the break. Furthermore, the supervisor may discuss what in their personal development the individual group members would like to focus on during the next term.

The supervisor and the group may also use the last session to check the attendance of group members during the past term. I tend to ask someone in the group to write on the board while I go through my notes: who have attended the supervision sessions, who have raised issues and which supervision questions and what themes have been covered at the supervision sessions? See diagram

Name	Attendance No. of sessions	Who has been in focus Mark who	Supervision question & issues from my notes

This helps the supervisor to write the certificate on how many hours each participant has attended. It also makes clear how the supervision time has been divided between group members, permitting a discussion on any uneven distribution such as: Why does certain individuals always have an issue they wish to raise, and others have barely raised one issue in a year? What can the supervisor and group members do specifically to enable all participants to be in focus? How can the supervisor help a supervisee who does not raise any issues?

Sometimes a participant has not raised any issue for several terms but has anyway been active in the supervision. It's important that the supervisor points this out. There is a difference of being in focus and not being in focus but always having something to say about someone else's professional work or how to act as a professional.

What could be evaluated?

Here follow some examples from different groups on how the supervisees express themselves in evaluations and feedback, based on what they will take away or have gained from the supervision. The supervisor could also focus on herself as supervisor: what has been good respectively less so, what should she maintain of what she is doing, what to remove or change?

These citations from some of my groups are divided into four categories, depending on what has been in focus:
- Evaluation aimed at the group
- Evaluation aimed at individual development – what did you gain from the supervision
- What you want to develop in yourself or as a group during next term
- Evaluation of the supervisor, supervision style and model.

The examples are taken from supervision at workplaces, but not from education-based supervision and presented as citations without comment. The citations may speak for themselves.

Evaluation focused on the group

"We've become a group, a good group."
"We got guidance. We've worked through the questions we had to deal with."

"We've got to know each other better. Done work on ourselves and on our professional role."

"There's warmth in the group. Tolerance. Now, we're quite close-knit. Became more confident in the group. We have fun together. There's no prestige. Everyone participates. Listens to one another. It's good we had the chance to work with the group. Good that we see our professional role clearly. By observing what we didn't know, we've become stronger as a group."

"We've learned how to set limits. Making sure we have clear assignments."

"I feel we know the individuals in the group. I'm never nervous beforehand – what will it be like today? When we use cards, everyone becomes more visible, we get more personal."

"The supervision group is fantastic – we have plenty of elbow room. Everyone has been generous in sharing their thoughts, what works and what doesn't work. There was openness and you could show vulnerability. You didn't need to think before speaking your mind – everyone takes it seriously."

"There is trust among colleagues. We understand each other better now and support one another. The supervision helps us as a group not to lose the perspective of the child."

"Everyone is involved – not passive, not just an audience. It's fine adding relevant theory sometimes."

"Everyone has been given space and taken space."

Evaluation of individual development

What did you get from the supervision?

"In the supervision the attention is on whom I am in the case work. I've learned much from my colleagues. The supervision helps giving me a broader picture. A new way of handling issues. There are many ways to proceed. Learning how to describe your challenges. I have learned self-reflection finding the answer myself."

"It takes time to formulate a supervision question. We had to look for and select an alternative. A previous supervision offered only one answer."

"You get tired of yourself – it's useful to hear the reflections of others. Test yourself. Challenge: what do I really want? "

"Gives me courage to ask questions to clients and colleagues."

"It's a challenge: you have to think hard – and stay alert."

"Looked at different ways of solving a problem. Leaving with new energy. Makes me vulnerable, but the supervision helps me in my encounters with the client."

"Missed several sessions. Attended too few sessions but each time has given me a lot. Learning by listening to matters presented by others. I take it on board. Means a lot that we may think in different ways, having different viewpoints. Testing and thinking so I don't think weirdly."

"Personally, my approach is permeated by the different qualities and personalities involved. What you are – the way you are. A positive girl relies on herself. I know it's hard sometimes, I also have several children. Reaching normality opens doors in difficult problems."

"I was taken aback by my sensitivity. Felt silly when I cried in the supervision session last time. The supervision brought up things in my past that I haven't dealt with in my life. It's about fleeing from other things in life. To realise how hard it is when you can't influence. Had to get out of the situation on my own. Putting words to it and understanding how difficult things can be is good sometimes."

"Tough process in the supervision, having to be in touch with one's own feelings. How to handle the situation. You examine yourself. It's a challenge to expose oneself in front of colleagues – not always easy."

"Using supervision, developing your tools – getting better at reaching the target group, better at collaboration. Feel more confident about how to talk to youths. Supervision is a time for pause when we can air our feelings."

"Process supervision is about understanding my feelings, figuring out – what's it about? The answers are not the most important, rather how to get there. Interaction, reflection, one's approach to the case. The supervision moves deeper, it awakens something in me; why do I get affected like that. Need to address my questions in depth. Finding a way to relate to what happens to me; my own reflections."

"Supervision has helped me to be clearer when encountering the client. Getting a better structure. You've summarised on the board, and we have taken photographs, so we bring this with us. Finding strategies, to pause and meet with others. Informative. Got to know my colleagues in a different way."

"The questions you asked made me go more in depth than I wanted. I don't know the effects of those questions. Now I understand how much trauma I am left to deal with from the war."

"To begin with I was always nervous. But it gave me tools. I've become clearer about myself. My patience when working on my cases was not always great. Became a little more strict and clearer about limits. I like the cards."

"Getting help arranging my thoughts for future conversations with the client. Don't remain in a feeling of frustration after the supervision. Getting tired but feel relief. We're encouraged to trust our own judgment."

What do you want to focus during the next semester?

Supervision groups usually run during six to eight semesters. It may be a good idea after two or three terms to ask every participant what he wants to focus on during the next semester. What do you wish to develop in yourself at the forthcoming sessions after the break? This is also a basic question the supervisor should keep in mind when someone is in focus in supervision. Some voices on this:

"Thinking more about what I do."

"Gaining more tools for the work. New thoughts, ideas."

"Working more on myself. Become wiser as a person. Not to be trapped."

"To be able to handle conflicts rather than escaping."

"Getting tools to be able to give the client tools."

"Supervision should be a challenge." "Challenging myself. We have power. Seeing my professional role more clearly."

"How can my knowledge be a resource?"

"Negotiate a reasonable course – finding better ways in my own work."

"Working in the supervision – how can I influence the structure at work. Working with my own structure – how I want to shape my professional role."

"Use the supervision to get on in my cases."

"The supervision helps me to land and to do things differently."

"Reflecting on what happens in the dialogue with the client. What did I do? What more needs to be done? We never have time to think and reflect at work."

"Chance to pause – to speak one's mind – also to get confirmation: you've done the right thing."

"Want more of a link to theory next term."

"Want you to help us to find our group spirit. Need your help to make us feel like a team. We are a team, we have goals. We need more time to listen to one another, that would improve my understanding of the others."

"We have to listen more to each other."

"We agree that we don't agree. We have no frames or any structure in our work."

When group members talk about what they want to have in focus we have a thorough dialogue on the topic. We also may discuss the format and how to proceed in order to reach what the individual or group wants to do.

Evaluation of supervisor, supervision style and model

As I wish all the group members to individually give me feedback both on me as a supervisor and my model, I categorise their replies in terms of what they say about:
a) my supervision style
b) what I should maintain as a supervisor
c) what I should change as a supervisor.

Supervision style

Even though I am here citing what the groups have said about my supervision style, it can also be seen in the replies what the groups expect from any supervisor. What is appreciated and how does it support them in their professional work.

"You stick to the framework and have a structure. This is a place for work."

"When you use the board, it becomes clear. We can go back and look at it while the supervision is going on. There are many thoughts that come up and then it's easy to miss something that has been said. But it's on the board. Excellent when you are using different colours. It makes it easier to see."

"You must work during the supervision. As a supervisor you notice – you intervene, ask more questions. We don't get away with anything. You are controlling the supervision. All the time you are bringing us back to what we're talking about. We must think twice. Answer questions. You are directing. Keeping things on course."

"A bit intimidating and challenging having to look closely at oneself. Good you have a softer side. You're straight, honest and challenging."

"You're open and share things. Having a broad knowledge. It can be troubling at times when you ask: 'What is your question?'"

"You don't forget things. The set-up you have is important. I do get attention, can relax. It's not possible to remain idle during the supervision. One must work here. You don't give up. One must think. You return. You structure the material. We are getting better results being active. We all must be active. You have a clear line, a structure. In the end it pays off, even if it's tough. The scheme means I can stand it."

"As a supervisor you ask: 'What happens to you here?' You always return to oneself."

"You create a permissive climate – we get support. Never been judged for what I think and feel. Could raise any issue."

"Differences are tolerated. It may turn personal but not awkward. Sometimes you challenge in a positive way. It took a while to understand what you are talking about when you ask questions."

"You dare to be embarrassing."

"You're curious, interested in the individual."

Discontent with the supervision

Sometimes there are group members who are not satisfied and want to break off the supervision. Here are some voices:

"Don't understand what you're doing?"

"Don't get much from the supervision. Thinking about other things during the supervision. Sometimes after the supervision, I am thinking I would have been better off staying at work and used my time more effectively."

"Felt stupid, incompetent when you ask questions I can't answer."

"Feeling afraid of you. It's unpleasant. Don't know what's expected of me. I get a pain in the belly when heading for the supervision."

"I don't want supervision from you but want to be part of the supervision. I learn a lot when others raise their issues."

"Feel like you are denouncing and don't consider that I did a good job."

"Your questions were tough to begin with. Felt a bit like an interrogation. Not used to being questioned in such depth."

"Your supervision doesn't suit us. Your way of asking questions. It's more suitable for people who are therapists. We're not therapists. We don't meet our clients that often."

"It felt like you wanted to end the supervision with us."

"The supervision feels like a strain and it's not much fun attending."

"I was nervous about coming to the supervision. Don't understand your questions or what you want. Wondered if I was stupid when I didn't understand. Didn't dare to ask."

"I don't want to look at what happens to me in meeting the client. Don't want to look at what I feel. I know it, but I don't care about that. I want a method, not the supervision you're offering."

I have noticed that such comments are more common now, than was the case fifteen years ago. The mobility of groups has changed. These days groups are more mobile, newly graduated are given very tough assignments and are asking for method supervision rather than process supervision. This makes it harder and tougher for the supervisor. There are many more supervisors, different directions, and the procurer primarily requests intervention methods.

If negative comments on the supervision are given within the time frame of a series of sessions, solutions can usually be found. I just need to adapt and relate differently to some individuals, or they get to know me better and realise that I'm not wishing to hurt or offend. Some individuals abstain after consultation with me and the manager, while others in the group who are satisfied with the supervision continue. Sometimes, what was said about me were really projections. Some individuals could see this, while others left the supervision. In almost all such cases, I have had a dialogue with the person who was not satisfied and wanted to leave. The dialogue was usually face to face and rewarding, both for me as a supervisor and for the person in focus. Both learned from the experience of doing this together. Both appreciated the opportunity to close the process in a constructive way.

I'm also interested in getting feedback on what I as a supervisor should maintain and what I may need to change. It does not automatically mean that I will modify my style, but if something appears to be recurrent, I must work on the problem in my meta-supervision.

What the supervisor may maintain and continue doing

"You use rewarding instructive methods and should keep doing that."
"You can take criticism, you don't dismiss it, that's good."
"We touch many different levels – processes in the supervision."
"It's good to be able to give feedback to the manager."
"It's been personal, but it hasn't been tough."
"Good when you ask: what is your question? How do you want to work?"
"As a supervisor, you're persistent. Asking in a positive way. I've learned from this and now ask my clients more questions than before. Get a clearer picture

and a better relationship. I challenge myself more now. The dialogues are on a deeper level. Using the board works well at a pedagogic level, I can see what we're talking about, don't have to keep it in mind – can focus on my own thoughts."

" You challenge me. You don't give up in your questions. They're on a deeper level. Can be annoying but good because I'm also good at being impulsive. Good to get reflections from colleagues. Had to think twice and reflect on my own actions. Cards and pictures are a good way to make us reflect on where we are now. Instead of just talking about where we are. Good to have picture cards as a starting point."

"How are you as a supervisor: it can be frustrating that you don't give up but for me it was good to slow down because I'm often in too much of a hurry."

"It's good that we don't decide on who is to raise an issue the next time."

"Continue as we've been doing."

"You should maintain your way of using the group, there's a basic structure, a focus on participation and attention. It's good that you write in different colours on the board."

"Good to do work on ourselves. Using the whole group. Forced to participate. The form is good, that we reflect, and you step in at the end."

"Good that you ask: 'How do you want to use the group? What do you want to get out of the group?'"

"Whoever is in focus for supervision decides how to use the group. Sometimes we don't have a supervision question, but just want to talk and unburden ourselves in the presence of someone who listens and is attentive. It feels good that I don't need a supervision question ready."

What the supervisor should change

"The start of the supervision has sometimes been too long. I got impatient and thought: 'Let's get going now.'"

"You might sometimes start by asking: 'What are the expectations for the day' – not just ask at the beginning when you interviewed us. We can then refer to conditions at work right now, or our expectation of the supervision today."

"The first time wasn't too great. You should have stopped us when we were just going on and acting the same in supervision as we do at work. We talk too much. It's a power struggle between us and that's also what happened in the supervision."

"Explain the framework of the supervision as carefully as possible so that all the participants understand. Maybe several times."

"Be more demanding about professionalism. Sharpen the presentation on the framework and say: 'Here you should forget about yourself, your private life and your experience.' Some would claim that their private experience is what helps them most to act in a professional way."

The various citations show that group members have very different expectations of the supervisor. In such a case it's necessary for the supervisor to be responsive, to listen and to be flexible.

7. Closing the supervision

A SUPERVISION ASSIGNMENT can be closed in many ways and for several reasons. Usually the assignment ends after five or six terms based on a mutual decision of the group and supervisor that it is time to change supervisor. If you as a supervisor have been active for a long time and led many groups, you have a lot of experience how to terminate your assignment.

In this section, I explain how the supervisor can end a supervision assignment. The several types of closure are categorised and described based upon whose initiative the supervision ends, how the assignment ends and why.

Closure of a supervision assignment may be the result of:

- a mutual agreement to close
  - after the period stated in the contract
  - before the contract period has ended
- on the group's initiative not to extend the contract period
- on the supervisor's initiative to close before the end of the contract period
- the organization is closing.

Agreement to close

Closing according to the contract

The supervision typically ends according to the contract which usually runs for one year at a time. It is the supervisor's responsibility to address whether the contract should be extended or not. I usually raise the issue of ending the supervision in the middle of the second term: "Should we finish after the current term or extend it for another year?" Thereby, both the supervisor and the supervision group have time to prepare for the closure of the supervision. At the final supervision session, I tend not to supervise at all, with the notion not to start off a process which won't be followed up, as it's the last meeting.

Closing before the end of the contract period

Sometimes I or the group choose to close a supervision assignment while the supervision is still ongoing, i.e. before the end of the contract period. The reasons for this may vary. A concrete situation: I supervised a group for five terms, and we decided to continue for another year. In this group several group members had left, and new members had joined. In the spring term, when we were discussing an extension for another year there was only one person present who had attended the supervision from the beginning. The other five had entered the group one by one and others had begun and left during the five terms. In the spring term to which I'm referring one new person had joined the group. Before the summer break we carried out an evaluation of the supervision.

We found that three out of the six individuals in the group had decided to leave to join other organizations in the autumn. Thus, three new supervisees who had not participated in selecting me as supervisor would remain in the group. Furthermore, during the autumn these three would move to other departments due to a planned reorganisation. We agreed that it would not be productive to maintain the supervision during the autumn as everything was in a state of flux, new persons would temporarily join the supervision two or three times out of five sessions during the term. We reflected on the situation together and decided that we should close the supervision. Those who remained with their new colleagues would look for a new supervisor during the autumn. In this context it was I as the supervisor who raised the issue of closing the supervision instead of carrying on. For this group it was the best solution. I had never met or spoken to the group manager and had no written agreement with her. All negotiations on the contract, hours and expectations was carried out with the group members only.

I have experience of a similar organization, but a completely different situation in which I had good contact with the group manager. Here, the manager together with me and the group decided that I would remain after the group members had been replaced and the organization underwent restructuring. During this process of change at work, we saw the value of the supervision providing a stable and secure meeting place for group members. When the situation in the organization had stabilized, we closed our supervision.

When a group terminates the contract

Sometimes, a group wishes to terminate the supervision because it has become a new group. Many new members have joined and selecting a new supervisor might be wise.

In a few instances I have hardly had time to set up the supervision when the group decides not to continue with me as supervisor. On one occasion the reason was that my supervision model was not useful to the group. They didn't have long, ongoing relationships with their clients and didn't think they would learn anything useful in the supervision, which includes reflection, an in-depth exploration of oneself on a personal as well as on a professional level and with clients. They would not have the same dialogue with their clients as we have in the supervision. The supervision felt like a burden and not great attending. The group became unresponsive and insecure. In the fourth and final meeting they spoke of attending supervision only to get a break from their demanding work and talk about the organization and about leadership. They also wanted to get to know each other better. They were a new group and had not yet had time to do this. My style of supervision is a challenge, and they were not yet ready for that, as a group they were not completely comfortable with each other. My questions and way of beginning the supervision session with cards was alien to them and they could not understand its meaning and purpose. Anyhow, we could close on a positive note where several issues were aired. There was an openness, and I shared my own feelings and my realisation that I should have done things differently from the beginning. In a way I think it's a pity we didn't work through the situation and learned together from the experience. It often happens that a client does not want to see the therapist or contact person but have no other choice. As a professional in supervision not wanting to attend could be a good starting point for reflection and dialogue trying to understand possible parallels. In such a situation a group discussion led by a person outside the organisation might be useful. If the supervision nevertheless is unproductive, it would at that point, of course, be terminated.

The supervisor's initiative to close the contract early

On very few occasions I, as the supervisor, have raised the subject of ending the supervision in the middle of the term. In such situations neither the group nor I have been satisfied with the process of the supervision. Our efforts have not led to any change. I witnessed how the group's dissatisfaction with the manager and atmosphere in the workplace shifted to express dissatisfaction with me and the atmosphere of the supervision, but I didn't have the right tools to tackle it. In this situation it would have been constructive if I had instead invited a moderator to lead the discussion, to help explore our process together with the group.

Whenever an organization will shut down

In Sweden during 2016 and 2017 a challenging situation arose in residential care homes for unaccompanied young migrants. I gave supervision in many places that eventually had to close. This was a theme in the supervision as I was aware of their imminent closure. Sometimes we have had to reduce the duration of the supervision. In all these places interaction with the manager was helpful in terminating the supervision. The managers willingly let the group discuss the changed situation and how they might discuss with the youths their changed conditions, due to new Swedish policies regarding unaccompanied young migrants. My book 'Att möta människor i trauma. Om ensamkommande unga' (Cajvert, 2018). (Meeting people in trauma: the unaccompanied youngster) covers this topic.

A group searches new supervisors during the supervision

For a long time, I have thought about the situation when a group, in the process of finishing with one supervisor, simultaneously also is looking for and interviewing new supervisors. It is complex. The group is for some time (at least one term) involved in two concurrent processes. I've noticed the level of commitment changing when this happens. There is less energy in the supervision sessions. More members are frequently absent from the supervision. There is greater focus on the work, visiting clients and at the same time searching and interviewing new potential supervisors. Sometimes group members want to cancel the final term of the supervision, especially if they are about to leave the organization.

These circumstances influence the group process, but also me as a supervisor. As supervisor I should keep the process alive, not being disturbed by changes in the group and trying to retain a meaningful and productive supervision for those who participate.

If the group decide to take a break after completing the supervision and not until then look for a new supervisor, each participant may during the final two sessions in dialogue with the supervisor express what he wants from the new supervision for his own development and as a group. When the group is aware of what it wants to develop, the discussion can help reflecting on what type of supervision might best fulfil these needs. When the group has clarified requirements and direction of the supervision, the group can move on to discuss how to interview prospective supervisors, and how to ask relevant questions about the supervisor's model, style, and theoretical affiliation. As a group it is a way of preparing for an interview with a new potential supervisor.

Ideally the group should finish the process with the current supervisor and take a break for a term while they look for a new supervisor. After several years with one supervisor it may also be wise not to have any supervision at all for one or two terms. The group can apply what they learned in the supervision and if necessary, supervise each other, a collegial supervision, as described in the next section. It can be helpful both for developing a collective spirit and to make use of each other's competence and experience.

Model for collegial supervision

This model is based on group members deciding beforehand on who should raise questions, who should function as supervisor, who should keep the record and who should give feedback to the acting supervisor. The model has distinct stages and gives clear instructions on who does what in each stage. Each stage has a clear content and a timeframe everyone should keep.

The supervisor's role is to maintain structure and the timetable. Making sure everyone understands which issue or dilemma the supervisee wants to explore, making sure questions raised by the other group participants are short and concise and answers address the question.

The recordkeeper is noting down the essence of the questions and how different group members frame their solutions. If previously agreed, the record is sent to the teacher responsible for the course.

The group member responsible for feedback to the supervisor follows the process and group dynamic. At the end of the supervision, he gives brief feedback to the supervisor on how the supervisor followed the structure and has responded to the supervisee and others in the group. He should be able to give concrete examples of what has been good (at least three things that the supervisor has done well) and argue why this has been good – what was the effect? Importantly, he should address what the supervisor could have done differently, one or two things. Here, too, should be argued and given suggestions on how that "otherwise" could be. It is important not only to give feedback but also to share your own idea of how you would do yourself and why.

Stage 1. Informative phase (max 15 min.)

In this phase the supervisee presents the issue, problem, dilemma, situation, or other matter that he wants to address in the group. He describes what type of help, support and focus he is looking for. The supervisor assists in making this clear for all, and the group can also ask factual questions for further clarifications. The supervisor ensures that group members ask concrete questions and do not give advice or ideas or dispute anything. One should not discuss the situation; the questions must be aimed at gaining clarity on the narrative and the issue. The questions are of an informative kind. Each group member asks one or two questions, and no more. The supervisee answers the questions without enlarging his narrative.

Stage 2. What is the supervisee's dilemma or issue? (max 10 min.)

What would I have done to try to solve or work with it?

In this phase each participant on her own writes down what she perceives as the essential aspect of the presentation. In other words: What is the dilemma or the issue? At this stage there is no discussion of what she wrote.

Each group member also writes down how he would solve the dilemma, situation, or issue if he faced the same problem.

Stage 3. Sharing (max 10 min.)

Each group member reads aloud what he has written. There should be no discussion. The supervisee in focus may ask questions if there is something that he does not understand or have not completely grasped. He should not question, not defend, or argue.

Stage 4. What does the supervisee learn? (max 10 min.)

At this stage the supervisee shares how he intends to resolve his dilemma or issue based on what he has heard. He might have gained inspiration to solve his issue by any of the proposed solutions or selects the one serving him best given the current situation. Only he can decide what will be the best approach. He may also, having listened to the others, produce a solution of his own.

Stage 5. Feedback to the supervisor (max 10 min.)

In this phase the observing group member gives feedback to the supervisor. She should report what has been positive, good, rewarding, and resourceful. She should argue for any new perspective or proposal of new ways to deal with similar situations. Other group members may also provide feedback and discuss the supervisor's resources.

Stage 6. Evaluation – what did each participant learn? (max 5 min)

At this stage everyone shares, briefly, what he will take home the session. What has each participant learned?

8. How to articulate your style of supervision?

IF THE SUPERVISOR WANTS to articulate ideas about her style of supervision, she might ask herself the following questions and reflect:

What is supervision? Clarifying this would help you to communicate your view of supervision to the groups you are meeting.

How would you describe yourself as a supervisor? You should be aware of what you are doing and how you are working as a supervisor. Observe yourself in different supervision settings. Engage in evaluation and ask the group to describe what you are doing. Also, ask for feedback on what you are doing.

What is important to yourself as a supervisor? Reflect on what you believe is important to know, communicate, take on board as a supervisor and how that should be conveyed to the supervision group. To be aware of how to use what you consider important in supervision.

What is a good supervision? Raise your awareness of your own idea of a good supervision. What happens then in the supervision? What constitutes a supervision session? How do you deal with various themes, questions, attitudes and behaviour of the individual and of the group?

Do you have a supervision style or model? How is this communicated to the group? Be aware of how to build relations and trust and handling the group process. What support do the supervisees get in their professional development?

What techniques and materials are used in the supervision? Awareness of why you use techniques and materials in the supervision is important. What do you want to achieve and influence? What are you allowed to influence?

How would the supervisees describe you as a supervisor? You should ideally be able to imagine how the supervisees may describe you as a supervisor. What would they say? To reflect on your own image and your perceptions of the images and ideas others might have of yourself may lead to greater self-knowledge and confidence. Be brave, test something new; dare to listen and take on board opinions and critical thoughts.

What theoretical orientation do you have as a supervisor? It's important to be aware of your own theoretical basis. The task of the supervisor is to help others to be aware of theoretical knowledge and how to apply it in practice. It helps the supervisee to behave professionally at work and to grow. If the supervisor does the same for herself, it becomes easier to help others to become aware of their professional skills. Knowing how you know what you know.

Which techniques are appealing to the supervisor? All techniques used by the supervisor are hopefully of use to the supervisee and the group in progressing in the process and to reach set goals. Knowing as a supervisor about the purpose of what you want to achieve helps you not to use your common sense or not having a goal. You do what you do with a purpose which is based on something, or on someone else's theories. This increases professionalism, gives professional self-confidence and trust in your knowledge and approach. An awareness that distinguishes the professional from the amateur, or others lacking the same education or theoretical background.

What do you want to continue to develop as a supervisor? What are you curious about? What would you like to develop in yourself and why? Something you want to develop based on your experience of how it worked in the supervision.

How do you get there? Start articulating what you need and then consider how to achieve that. What further training is needed? Meta-supervision? Which direction do you choose and why? Do you need therapy? It's about taking responsibility for your own ongoing development, on a professional and personal level.

What do you need from others, and which others, to reach your set goals? Which others do you need to reach the goals you have set for yourself? Employers, colleagues, your own family? To become aware of how they can help you to reach the set goals; to develop.

Closing words –
importance of using process supervision

Through process supervision the individual's understanding of his own feelings and thoughts increases. In turn, this establishes preconditions for professional and personal growth and development. In process supervision and working with the group members, an open problem-solving climate is created that builds confidence and trust between the group members, for example, by understanding the tensions that might occur between them, and possibly the leader and organisation, due to age, gender, opinions and cultural background. Working with process supervision and interactive processes promotes the individual's and the group's maturity and health and provides constructive change. Individual freedom of thought and expression is valued, along with spontaneity and an openness to change. This freedom to express one's thoughts and feelings creates an opportunity for the group to become more close-knit, to find alternative types of behaviour and a professional attitude. This happens when the supervisee asks questions such as "How should I respond to this demanding client?", "How should I respond to the troublesome, irascible man?" or "How can I get through to this child?"

Process supervision focusing the therapist's thoughts and feelings creates an awareness of your own attitudes, prejudices, values and blind spots that may otherwise cause disruption in encounters with vulnerable groups. Recognizing a need for a different approach leads to a more humane and compassionate attitude, seeing the need of vulnerable persons for help and support.

The group spirit developing in supervision and the creation of a positive climate of trust help the individual member to reduce his loneliness and isolation through meaningful contact with others in the group. This experience creates energy and can be communicated to the client.

Process supervision for professionals does not provide a solution to the supervisees' work situation. Process supervision gives the supervisees the opportunity to get to know themselves as professionals, to express their feelings and thoughts and their frustration in specific situations that requires a different approach, not to affect the clients. The professionals can gain knowledge and tools so that both themselves and the group find new perspectives and resources to understand and deal with their situation. Rogers (1976) writes about the future and the changes we will be faced with: "What we really need is not changed institutions, but change built into the life of the institutions: an instrument for continuous renewal of organisational forms, structure and planning" (p. 178).

In process supervision the feelings and thoughts of group members are emphasised 'here and now' – initially without any analysis or explanation. It creates a space to express precisely what matters *now* without being questioned, condemned, denied or diminished. The approach of the supervisor and group of being open, daring to express their feelings without fear of being offended or judged, I would argue leads to, as Rogers describes the members of the group "developing in a climate of freedom and support to becoming more spontaneous, more flexible, closer to their feelings, more open to their experiences, more expressive and trusting in their interpersonal relationships" (Rogers, 1976 p. 181).

Providing the opportunity for this type of group process may create expectations in the individual and in the organization. The group becomes aware of its core values and ethics and how these affect every meeting and any work with a vulnerable target group in need of professional help, and an understanding of the demanding situation in which individuals finds themselves. Awareness of his own experiences generates insight in each group member.

Supervision should lead to a new continuity so group members may develop a relationship and mutual confidence in one another, and in the supervisor.

Supervision should be predictable and offer an opportunity for development and learning. It helps group members to develop their competence as a group and to support one another. Such a development strengthens an organization and supports the professional work with the target group.

References

Anderson, H. & Goolishian, H. A. (1992). *Från påverkan till medverkan. Terapi med språksystemiskt synsätt.* [From influence to participation. Therapy in a language system perspective] Stockholm: Mareld.

Belin, S. (1993). *Vansinnets makt. Parallellprocesser vid arbete med tidigt störda and psykotiska patienter.* [The power of madness. Parallel processes in work with early disturbed and psychotic patients] Stockholm: Natur & Kultur.

Bernard, J. M. & Goodyear, R. K. (2009). *Fundamentals of Clinical Supervision.* 4th edition. Upper Saddle River, New Jersey, Columbus, Ohio: Pearson Education.

Bernler, G. & Johnsson, L. (1985). *Supervision i psykosocialt arbete.* [Supervision in psychosocial work] Stockholm: Natur & Kultur.

Bernler, G., Cajvert, L., Johnsson, L. & Lindgren, H. (1999). *Psykosocialt arbete, idéer and metoder.* [Psychosocial work, ideas and methods] Stockholm: Natur & Kultur.

Bie, K. (2012). *Reflektionshandboken.* [Handbook of reflection] Malmö: Gleerups.

Bion, W. R. (1961). *Experiences in groups and other papers.* Social science paperbacks. London: Tavistock Publications.

Bobacken, B. & Pålsson, K. (2012). *Bättre teamkänsla! med Teamkort. Sån är jag ... och du?* [Better team spirit! with Teamcard. I am such ... and you?] Jönköping: Ledning & Ledarskap AB.

Buber, M. (1990). *Det mellanmänskliga.* [Interpersonal relations] Ludvika: Dualis Förlag.

Cajvert, L. (1998). *Behandlarens Kreativa Rum: Om handledning.* [The therapist's creative room. On supervision] Lund: Studentlitteratur.

Cajvert, L. (2011). A model for dealing with parallel processes in supervision.

Journal of Social Intervention: Theory and Practice – 2011 – Volume 20, Issue 1, pp. 41- 56. URN:NBN:NL:Ul:10-1-101308.

Cajvert, L. (2013). Handledning : Behandlarens kreativa rum.[Supervision – the therapist's creative room] Lund: Studentlitteratur.

Cajvert, L. (2016). *Studentsupervision under verksamhetsförlagd utbildning.* [Student supervision in clinical practice] Lund: Studentlitteratur.

Cajvert, L. (2018). *Att möta människor i trauma. Om ensamkommande unga.* [To meet someone in trauma: the unaccompanied youngster] Lund: Studentlitteratur.

Casement, P. (1986). *Att lära av patienten. En granskning av interaktionen mellan terapeut and patient and dess betydelse för den psykoterapeutiska processen.* [An investigation of the therapist-patient interaction and its importance in the psychotherapeutic process] Stockholm: Wahlström & Widstrand.

Eide, T. & Eide, H. (2012). *Kommunikation i praktiken – relationer, samspel and etik inom socialt arbete, vård and omsorg.* [Communication in practice – relations, interplay and ethics in social work and care] Malmö: Liber.

Evang, A. (1991). *Personlighet and borderline.* [Personality and borderline] Stockholm: Natur & Kultur.

Gordan, K. (1998). *Psykoterapisupervision inom utbildning, i kliniskt arbete och på institution.* [Supervision of psychotherapy in education, clinical work and at institutions] Stockholm: Natur & Kultur.

Gunnarsson, S. (2014). *Professionell feedback. Medvetna mötens magi. Om konsten att förbättra prestation, arbetsklimat, skapa utveckling and nå uppsatta mål. Konsten att be om and ge feedback.* [Professional feedback. The magic of mindful meetings. On the art of improving performance, work climate, creating development and reaching set aims. The art of asking for and giving feedback] Bromma: Gunnarssons Förlag.

Hawkins, P. & Shohet, R. (2000). *Supervision in the helping professions.* Maidenhead: Open University Press.

Igra, L. (1988). *På liv och* död. Om destruktivitet *och livsvilja*. [Life and death. On destructiveness and desire to live] Stockholm: Natur & Kultur.

Kellermann, P. F. (1992). *Focus on psychodrama. The therapeutic aspects of psychodrama.* London: Jessica Kingsley Publishers Ltd.

Kordeš, U. (2008). Fenomenološko istraživanje [Phenomenological research]. I N. Koller-Trbovic & A. Žižak (red.), *Kvalitativni pristup u društvenim znanostima [Qualitative approach to social sciences]* (s. 55–73). Zagreb: Edukacijsko – rehabilitacijski fakultet.

Korman, H. & Söderquist, M. (1994). *"Snacka om mirakel!" En bok om samarbete med missbrukare and deras nätverk.* [" Talk about a miracle!" A book on collaboration with addicts and their network] Stockholm: Mareld.

Löwenborg, C. (2013, 2016, 2017). *Om konkreta, visuella and gestaltande metoder i supervision.* [On concrete, visual and configuring methods in supervision] Laholm: Tryckpunkten.

Nilsonne, Å. (2017). *Processen. Möten, mediciner, beslut. En professionell självbiografi.* [The process, meetings, therapies, decisions. A professional autobiography Stockholm: Natur & Kultur. '

Ogden, T. (1987). *Projektiv identifikation and psykoterapeutisk teknik.* [Projective identification and psychotherapeutic technique] Stockholm: Natur & Kultur.

Rogers, C. (1976). *Människor i grupp. Om encounter groups – vart de syftar and hur de fungerar –* (W & W-serien 359). [On encounter groups] Stockholm: Wahlström & Widstrand.

Soltvedt, M. (2005). *BOF – Barnorienterad familjeterapi.* [Child centred family therapy] Falun: Mareld.

Thylefors, I. (2016). *Chef- and ledarskap inom välfärdsorganisationer.* [Head- and leadership in welfare organizations] Stockholm: Natur & Kultur.

Tähkä, V. (1987). *Psykoanalytisk psykoterapi*. [Psychoanalytical psychotherapy] Stockholm: Natur & Kultur.

Ullman, M. (1996). *Att förstå drömmens språk*. [Understanding the language of a dream] Stockholm: Natur & Kultur.

Van Kessel, L. & Haan, D. (1993). The intended way of learning in supervision seen as a model. *The Clinical Supervisor, 11*(1), 29–43.

Wittgenstein, L. (1978). *Filosofiska undersökningar*. [Philosophical investigations] Stockholm: Bonniers.

Wonnacott, J. (2012). Mastering Social Work Supervision. London and Philadelphia: Jessica Kingsley Publishers.

Young, J: Klosko, J. & Weishaar, M. (2003). *Schema therapy. A practioner's guide*. New York: Guildford Publications.

Žorga, S. (2002). Supervision: the process of life-long learning in social and educational professions. *Journal of Interprofessional Care, 16*(3), 265–276.

Milton Keynes UK
Ingram Content Group UK Ltd.
UKHW020646041223
433752UK00018B/1164